Psychogenic Polydipsia:

Treatment Strategies and Housing Options

Dr. Donald Hutcheon R.Psych.,
C.Psychol. (UK)

Psychogenic Polydipsia: Treatment Strategies and Housing Options
by Dr. Donald Hutcheon

© 2012

ACFEI Media
2750 E. Sunshine
Springfield, MO 65804

ISBN: 978-0-9832601-4-1

Printed in the United States. First printing

ACKNOWLEDGEMENTS

I wish to thank my parents who gave me the drive to achieve and succeed. I also owe a debt of gratitude to my wife and two sons for their support throughout the completion of the book! My brother in Calgary, whose courage and tenacity of living with a severe disability has contributed to my understanding of "dignity of risk". Ernie Cameron, whose kindness and support towards my brother and father was inspirational. I thank Dr. Arnold Abramson, who worked so diligently on the graphs and diagrams, and Ed Peaco, who did a superb editing job. Lastly, Dr. Don Pazaratz, my friend and ally throughout my 40-year career. He is a Canadian authority in residential treatment services for adolescents and a wonderful inspiration.

BIOGRAPHY

Dr. Hutcheon has been a senior psychologist for the past 10 years at Riverview Psychiatric Hospital in Coquitlam, a suburb of Vancouver, British Columbia. From 2001-2006 he was the attending psychologist assigned to Riverview Hospital's "Water Ward" for those patients diagnosed with psychogenic polydipsia.

In the past, Dr. Hutcheon has held posts as Vice President then Treasurer of the British Columbia Psychological Association (2004-2008). Other previous positions have included Director of Residential Services for the Vocational Rehabilitation Resources Institute (VRRI) in Calgary, Alberta, (1985-1986) and supervising the Child Abuse Hotline of Alberta (1982-1985). This unit was the prototype for the "Kids Line" of Canada, a National emergency telephone center for victims of child abuse and neglect.

More recently, Dr. Hutcheon was Manager of the Young Physically Disabled Program (YPDP), an acquired brain injury rehabilitation inpatient unit at Dr. Vernon Fanning Chronic Care Hospital, Calgary, Alberta (1988-1995) and a partner in a Calgary-based private practice, Roberts, Hutcheon, and Howard Associates (1996-2001). During this period he became qualified as a chartered psychologist in the United Kingdom and also licensed in the Northwest Territories/Nunuvut in Canada's far north (2001).

In 2004 he co-wrote the prototype for the Canadian Psy.D curriculum, which was ratified by the CPA, and was a member of the BCPA Task Force on prescription privileges for psychologists in British Columbia (2009-2011). For the past 10 years, Dr. Hutcheon has operated a part-time private practice/consulting business in Port Coquitlam, specializing in mood/affect disorder, couples and family therapy, sport performance/outcome and industrial-organizational psychology. More recently he has consulted in parental assessment and child custody assessments in Northern Canada.

CONTENTS

CHAPTER THREE   63
BEHAVIORAL MANAGEMENT PRINCIPLES AND PROCEDURES:
STAFF TRAINING DOCUMENT (MODULES I – VI)

CHAPTER FIVE   163
RESIDENTIAL SETTINGS: A CONTINUUM OF CARE FOR CLIENTS DIAGNOSED WITH PSYCHOGENIC POLYDIPSIA

INTRODUCTION

The expressed purpose of the book is to provide an in-depth overview of recent treatment programs for psychogenic polydipsia from both an inpatient and outpatient perspective. The book details the treatment of psychogenic polydipsia from a biopsychosocial perspective, emphasizing behavioral management and psychosocial treatment interventions. The actual community-based treatment continuum is saved for the last chapter and describes a cogent group home residential model. More specifically and in order of level of care, highest to lowest:

1. Secure residential treatment group home (SRTGH);

2. Post-acute (intermediate) treatment group home (PAIT);

3. Residential treatment home (RTH);

4. Supported independent living facility (SIL);

5. Crisis respite resources (CRR).

It must be emphasized that community-based treatment for this dual-diagnosed clinical population, arranged in a continuum of service provision, is not unique. However, comprehensive descriptions of the design and working features of each phase of the group-home model have not been forthcoming from a review of literature.

It is this paucity of information regarding a viable treatment model in the community for clients diagnosed with psychogenic polydipsia that the idea of writing this book originated.

Chapter One:
Designing a Residential Continuum for Clients Diagnosed with Psychogenic Polydipsia

This chapter discusses in detail the nature of psychogenic polydipsia and its cause and effect on a diagnosed client. Other frequently used terms are provided to acquaint the uniformed reader, or to reacquaint the reader already experienced, but not directly involved with this clinical population. Client-care requirements are discussed regarding persons with severe and persistent mental illness, which requires services well above those provided at a secondary level of care. Risk factors are discussed from both a historical and more current perspective, supported by literature reviewed on behavioral programs for this clinical population.

Chapter Two:
A Comparison of Treatment Programs for Psychogenic Polydipsia

Nine different inpatient and outpatient treatment programs (1992-2006) are compared. Each program is described with the following headings to increase consistency and ease of reading: Preamble; Treatment; Results; Discussion. Lastly, a vision and mission statement is provided regarding a treatment program of which the author was personally involved (2001-2006).

Chapter Three:
Behavioral Management Principles and Procedures Staff Training Document (Modules I-VI)

This chapter describes in detail behavioral management principles that have been used to train a multidisciplinary team to effectively implement a behavioral management program with this unique and perplexing clinical population.

- Module 1 contains a pre-test quiz regarding knowledge of behavior modification principles, which is followed by a discussion of the normalization philosophy and writing integrated plans of care.
- Module 2 discusses operationalizing behavioral management terms, which include time, frequency, rate, accuracy, and criterion. In conjunction, developing long and short-term goals are discussed in detail.
- Module 3 describes behavioral assessments and issues in measuring and recording behavior and choosing measurements, recording and reporting procedures.
- Module 4 describes behavioral management procedures to successfully operationalize a treatment program using this method of intervention.
- Module 5 describes maintenance and generalization of behavior.
- Lastly, Module 6 includes the post-test quiz (repeat from pretest Module 1) and evaluation and adaptation procedures.

Chapter Four:
Psychosocial Rehabilitation as It Pertains to Psychogenic Polydipsia

A discussion unfolds about the principles, values and implementation of a psychosocial re-habilitation/re-adaptation program for clients diagnosed with schizophrenia and psychogenic polydipsia. A discussion of the psychological risk factors precipitated by psychogenic polydip-sia preambles a description of a psychosocial rehabilitation model, for clients with episodic self-induced water intoxication (SIWI). In conjunction, a number of important features of the psychosocial treatment model are discussed, which include: the integration of a behavioral management approach as components of a psychosocial treatment plan; the assessment of program effectiveness; the relationship between staffing ratios and the effectiveness of inpatient psychiatric units treating clients diagnosed with psychogenic polydipsia; and a recent model of psychosocial intervention for clients diagnosed with psychogenic polydipsia.

Chapter 5:
Residential Settings: A Continuum of Care for Clients Diagnosed with Psy-chogenic Polydipsia

This chapter describes the organization, design, and composition of the various group home facilities within a continuum of outpatient care. Subsequently, a description of factors regard-ing the administration of *a group home program for clients diagnosed with psychogenic poly-dipsia* is presented. This is followed by a section on treatment plans for clients diagnosed with psychogenic polydipsia, detailing the factors recommended for community day-treatment pro-gramming.

In addition, the section entitled "A group home continuum to treat psychogenic polydipsia" describes the makeup of the physical settings and staffing accommodation requirements for the continuum of group homes.

Lastly, a description of the group home/treatment continuum is described in detail regarding each phase of treatment: a staffing model that works; the admission and discharge criteria; the dual role of the outreach team; staffing and resident requirements to correspond with the suc-cessful treatment of psychogenic polydipsia; and a description of the crisis respite resources unit, for those residents who have decompensated in times of crisis and require emergency housing.

This is a detailed, comprehensive book and hopefully provides most of the relevant answers the reader may require concerning the establishment of a community-based treatment model for this clinical population.

CHAPTER ONE

Designing A Residential Continuum for Clients Diagnosed with Psychogenic Polydipsia

◇◇

PREAMBLE

Much is asked of a community residential program for clients diagnosed with a co-occurrent disorder (e.g., schizophrenia and psychogenic polydipsia). The respective group homes in such a continuum are designed to replicate, as close as possible, a "homelike" atmosphere for their residents. They must also create a rewarding milieu in which to be employed, deliver services competently to an often difficult and perplexing clientele, and present themselves as respected members of their communities. A community service program commences with the interaction of professionals and clientele with common interests, needs, or purposes. The staff involved will need to acquire specialized, clinical information and commit time and energy to make each segment of the group home continuum operational, with a view to increasing the skill set of its clientele. In this regard, the book presumes a reading population that is somewhat familiar with excessive fluid ingestion (i.e., psychogenic polydipsia) by psychiatric inpatients. To clarify any misunderstandings in terminology, the following information is presented to reacquaint the reader.

Psychogenic polydipsia is, on a continuum, the need-compulsion to seek out and overdrink any/all fluids and is a type of polydypsia exhibited by patients with mental illness and/or the developmentally disabled. It is present in a subset of schizophrenics. These individuals, often chronic schizophrenics with a long history of illness, frequently exhibit enlarged ventricles and shrunken cortex on MRI, making the physiological mechanism difficult to isolate from the psychogenic. Psychogenic polydipsia is a serious disorder and often leads to institutionalization as it can be very difficult to manage outside the inpatient setting. It should be taken very seriously and can be life threatening, as serum sodium is diluted to an extent that seizures and cardiac arrest can occur. Those individuals afflicted have been known to seek fluids from any source possible. The clinical presentation is as follows: the client drinks large amounts of any/all fluids, which raises the pressure of the extracellular medium. As a side effect, the antidiuretic hormone level is lowered. The urine produced by these clients will have a low electrolyte concentration, and it will be produced in large quantities (polyuria). If the individual is institutionalized, close monitoring by staff is necessary to control fluid intake. In extreme episodes, the client's kidneys will be unable to deal with the fluid overload, and weight gain will be noted (Gibson, WikiDoc Resources, 2010).

Polydipsia is increased thirst and excessive fluid intake, greater than 3 L per day. As many as 20% of schizophrenics are polydipsic and approximately 3.5%-5% of all schizophrenic clients develop the more serious syndrome of self-induced water intoxication (SIWI).

Compulsive water drinking: Individuals diagnosed with "psychogenic polydipsia," of which 80% are diagnosed with schizophrenia; have a fluid intake that is usually 4-10 L/day, some drink up to 22 L/day.

Hyponatremia: A low serum sodium level which is below 130 mmol/L (normal range 135-145 mmol/L).

Polyuria: Urine output in excess of 3 L/day. In the psychiatric population, polyuria exists as a compensatory mechanism for polydipsia; 25% of polydipsic clients have acute development of hyponatremia where there is a precipitous drop in serum sodium. This occurs sporadically and unpredictably and results in the syndrome of water intoxication.

Clozapine: An atypical antipsychotic medication, which, in low doses, is the most common pharmacological intervention in the treatment of self-induced water intoxication (SIWI). The restriction of fluid intake appears to have little or no influence on the excessive urge to drink by clients diagnosed with psychogenic polydipsia. As a result, investigators have turned to pharmacological interventions to treat either the polydipsia itself or the hyponatremia. Of Note: Clozapine has well-known side effects, including orthostatic hypotension, lowering of seizure threshold, anticholingeric toxicity, and significant incidence of agranulocytosis (1%-2%). Many clients with polydipsia or hyponatremia may have multiple physical illnesses that could preclude the use of clozapine (Verghese, de Leon & Josiassen, 1996).

Behavioral strategies: These include limiting the daily water intake when indicated, initiating fluid restriction when there is a significant weight increase, taking serum sodium levels if signs and symptoms of intoxication start to appear, providing constant attention for the client or locking the client in seclusion. Behavioral management programs should be mandatory.

Psychosocial rehabilitation (PSR): Programs for individuals diagnosed with psychogenic polydipsia, requiring tertiary care, should be guided by the principles of psychosocial rehabilitation (PSR) with sophisticated medication management and behavioral interventions. The PSR approach to service delivery is based upon eight fundamental and interconnected concepts (Bachrach, 1992):

1. Emphasizes the need for individually tailored interventions;

2. Either the individual's capacities be adapted to environmental realities or the environment be changed to suit the capacities of the person;

3. Oriented to exploitation of people's strengths;

4. Aims at the restoration of hope;

5. Emphasizes the vocational potential of mentally ill individuals;

6. Programs extend beyond work activities to encompass a full array of social and recreational life concerns;

7. Individuals are actively involved in their own care;

8. Is an ongoing process.

Awareness of polydipsia, polyuria, and hyponatremia dates back to the early part of the 20th century (Rowntree, 1923; Hoskins, 1933; Pfister, 1934; Sleeper, 1936; Miller, 1936). By modern standards these early studies were limited in methodology, and from a prepharmacological era make it clear that polydipsia and certain interrelated phenomena were seen in a significant fraction of chronic psychotic clients and that this disturbance of water regulation was clearly not a side effect of medication. Over 50 years later and in support of this statement, Vieweg, Rowe, Wampler, Burns & Spradlin (1989) showed that under normal conditions the body weight in healthy individuals did not increase by more than 1.2% in one day, whereas clients with chronic schizophrenia showed more than a 4% daily weight gain on average. Of Note: With this fall in serum sodium, symptoms may increase over time, or clients may be asymptomatic and then suddenly convulse.

CLIENT CARE REQUIREMENTS

Tertiary care is generally provided to persons with severe and persistent mental illness (SPMI).

These individuals exhibit conditions and problem behaviors that require services well above those provided at the secondary care level (Wasylenki, Goering, Cochrane, Simon & Wirth-Cauchon, 2000). This enriched type of treatment should require referral from secondary care for those individuals with problems that are complex and refractory to primary and secondary care. Criteria for success usually includes the need for higher levels of management and security, staff expertise, and staff and program resources, all in conjunction with more detailed and specialized assessment and treatment.

During the past 10 years, psychiatric service delivery research and expert opinion has successfully promoted community-based services providing tertiary care, to reduce reliance on traditional hospital-based tertiary care (Wasylenki et al. 2000). In contrast to past reliance on inpatient settings for tertiary care, it is possible to employ flexible strategies to maximize time in the least restrictive settings (Wasylenki et al. 2000). Level of staff expertise is a critical element of tertiary care. Tertiary care providers have generally advanced training and a commitment to service the population of clients with psychogenic polydipsia. Many long-term residents diagnosed with psychogenic polydipsia who reside in a provincial or state psychiatric hospital can graduate from inpatient tertiary care services to a community resource, if the funding allows for an appropriate staffing model. More specifically, hospital patients who have complex but stable conditions can be supported in community settings with access to tertiary services.

RISK FACTORS, CONSUMER PROFILE AND TREATMENT APPROACHES

In 1938 Barahal documented the first case of water intoxication in a client with schizophrenia. In 1974 Raskind reported a fatality from self-induced water intoxication. Vieweg, David, Rowe, Wampler, Burns, Spradlin (1985) subsequently reviewed 60 consecutive records of patients who died before the age of 53 years in a state hospital. Twenty-seven of those patients (45%) had a schizophrenic disorder, and of those 27 patients, five (18.5%) died from complications of SIWI. Deaths related to complications of SIWI remain a non-negligible and ignored cause of mortality in psychiatric populations. In regards to the tertiary treatment of this disorder, developing a "best practice" model for care is essential for increased quality of life for this clinical population. This includes the movement along a continuum of living arrangements, from secure hospital inpatient wards to residential facilities in the community with access to tertiary care as required.

During the 1980s and 90s, a trend towards community care of patients with psychiatric illnesses was developing, including, more recently, the residential care of clients diagnosed with severe and persistent mental illness (Eastern Oregon Human Services Consortium, 2010). A community based, residential continuum for clients diagnosed with psychogenic polydipsia will be examined in Chapter 5.

Excessive fluid drinking may occur in almost any psychiatric disorder (e.g., histrionic personality disorder). However, most cases (about 80%) of psychogenic polydipsia with self-induced water intoxication, occur in clients with a psychotic illness, usually of the schizophrenic type. The prevalence of compulsive water drinking in state psychiatric hospitals in the United States has been estimated between 7% and 18% (Jose & Perez-Cruet, 1979), and about half of this population suffer from the complications of SIWI (Hariprasad, Eisinger & Naider, 1980).

The cause of polydipsia remains unclear. Although there is some agreement in common areas of diagnosis and treatment interventions (e.g., clozapene, behavior modification, psychosocial rehabilitation), a consistent treatment approach throughout the years has included PSR strategies (i.e., psycho-education), which have been implemented in various tertiary care settings.

Almost 25 years ago Leiberman & Phipps (1987) developed a series of psycho-educational modules to teach social and instrumental skills. Several years later it was recommended that psychiatrists work with multidisciplinary teams in applying PSR approaches and that key elements be established in relation to the psychiatrist's role. These included providing expertise in psychiatric assessment and medication management; establishing, developing, and maintaining the therapeutic alliance with SPMI individuals; attending to the various interfaces between assessment and medication management; and the development of therapeutic alliances and rehabilitation interventions (Links, Kirkpatrick & Whelton, 1994).

Patients with severe mental illness require complex, specialized care and the development of a sophisticated medical management program. Clozapine has had a marked impact, with some individuals exhibiting behavioral problems as a result of psychogenic polydipsia, but the drug requires carefully developed strategies and close monitoring of its medication side effects (Essocks, Hargreaves & Dohm, 1996). Many patients with SPMI diagnosed with psychogenic polydipsia have cognitive deficits, which limit their ability to acquire or refine skills in rehabilitation programs. These deficits may include problems with distractibility and memory, lack of vigilance, attentional deficits, and limitations in planning and decision making. Although antipsychotic agents (e.g., clozapine) may have some impact on these deficits, complementary strategies based on behavioral approaches to cognitive rehabilitation are required. In the late 1990s, Silverstein, Hitzel & Schenkel (1998) identified interventions they felt would be effective in tertiary settings. Clients worked towards specified goals (e.g., reduced fluid consumption) through the reinforcement of successive steps. Using approaches such as token economies and PSR semi-weekly groups, team members rewarded small approximations of desired behaviors (e.g., reduced water drinking tendencies). In regard to the behavioral management strategies developed for the clinical population diagnosed with psychogenic polydipsia, the following section highlights its evolution.

LITERATURE REVIEW ON BEHAVIORAL PROGRAMS

The earliest case report (Klonoff & Moore, 1984) regarding behavioral interventions with clients diagnosed with psychogenic polydipsia was a response prevention and differential reinforcement with a 24-year-old man who complained of "desperate diuretic urge." Baseline fluid ingestion was 13 L per day. Biofeedback-assisted relaxation training was used to teach coping skills to reduce feelings of distress that accompanied the urge to overdrink. Fluid intake monitored by staff was the dependent variable. Following a 50-day hospitalization, the resident decreased fluid consumption 1-2 L Daily, and this reduction remained unchanged during a one-year follow-up.

The cornerstone of treatment strategies quickly became the regulation of fluid intake (Shesser & Smith, 1985; Viewig, David, Rowe, Peach, Veldhuis, Kaiser & Spradlin, 1985; Ledochowski, Kahler, Diensil, Hacker & Burns, 1988; Rinard, 1989). In conjunction, psycho-education (Baier, Robinson, DeShey, & Snider, 1989) was introduced to assist clients in assuming control over negative behavior manifesting the need for excessive water intake. Clients were provided the opportunity to discuss why fluid intake restrictions were needed, clarifying ideas about the necessity for fluid restriction and providing explanation in behavioral terms of the consequences of water intoxication and the recognition of symptoms such as increased irritability and demanding behavior.

Another objective of psycho-education was to assist clients in developing a sensitivity and awareness about negative behaviors (descrimitive stimuli) that trigger excessive water intake, in order to gain control of these behaviors.

The first behavioral interventions using a target weight procedure for psychogenic polydipsia was reported by Goldman and Luchins (1987). In their work, baseline weights and simultaneous serum sodium (i.e., blood/salt) concentrations were obtained twice a week for two weeks. A baseline mean weight and a mean serum sodium concentration were calculated and then used to predict a target weight that would be roughly equivalent to a plasma sodium level of 125 mEq/L. Eight subjects were weighed three times a week and whenever staff suspected water intoxication. If the weight exceeded the target weight, a serum sodium level was drawn. If the value was less than the minimum allowable, the subject was placed in seclusion for 24 hours but was allowed to eat, drink small amounts, and smoke. The subject was weighed every eight hours on the day of release and then returned to the previous schedule. Subsequent to the Goldman et al. (1987) article, many authors recommended monitoring the client's weight (Ashby, 1987; Cosgray, Hanna, Davidhizar & Smith, 1990; Lapierre, 1990; Snider & Boyd,1991) and serum sodium levels (Cosgray et al. 1990; Rinard, 1989; Snider & Boyd, 1991).

Bowen, Glynn, Barringer, Kurth & Hayden (1990) implemented a treatment and follow-up study of a 35-year-old female with chronic paranoid schizophrenia who, over a period of several years, had a history of multiple seizures secondary to polydipsia and water intoxication. The active treatment, conducted over 23 months in a psychiatric state hospital inpatient unit, involved multiple daily weights, fluid restriction, a variety of reinforcers for compliance of the program, and the use of locked time-out following significant weight gain or other specified violations of the program. During the client's final six months on the unit, a maintenance phase was implemented wherein most contingencies were faded. There was no reported recurrence of the problem 18 months after community placement. The eventual fading of contingencies, long-term follow-up, and involvement of a chronic schizophrenic client were unique features of this case report of behavioral treatment for polydipsia.

More specifically, six program violations were defined:

1. 5 lbs or greater weight gain in any 24-hour period,

2. Refusal to be weighed,

3. Unauthorized presence in a bathroom without escort (discontinued after 18 months),

4. Drinking from an unauthorized source (discontinued in the 19th month),

5. Leaving the dining room during a meal unattended (discontinued in the 19th month), and

6. Failure to terminate drinking at a water fountain after 20 seconds when prompted (initiated in the 14th month and discontinued in the 19th month).

About the same time, Delva and Cramer (1988) found that weight gain was a direct indicator of fluid/electrolyte balance. They recommended using body weight measurement for preventing water intoxication by establishing a target weight (7% above a basal weight) and weighing the individuals throughout the day. Once the target weight was reached, drinking was restricted. This data was supported by Koczapski, Ibraheem, Ashby, Pare, Jones & Ancell (1987) who found that recurrent afternoon fluid overload and dilutional hyponatremia were controlled through monitoring diurnal weight variation. Their results showed the usefulness of weight monitoring in the "early" diagnosis of water intoxication, as well as supporting target weight procedures as a reasonable intervention.

Baier & Gaertner (1991) stated that monitoring diurnal weight changes as a direct measure of fluid balance was promising in the prevention of water intoxication and maintenance of normal fluid balance. However, Vieweg and Leadbetter (1990) felt weight monitoring presented a clinical problem related to the reliability of the weights. In their study, they discussed the difficulty in establishing an accurate baseline weight. More specifically, individuals with disordered water balance often have compromised urinary tracts and can retain more than 3 L of urine. Thus, establishing a baseline weight without the validation of serum specimens could potentially lead to an elevated baseline. Catheterization would not eliminate the excessive fluid that is sometimes retained interstitially.

In contrast, the St. Louis State Hospital Target Weight Procedure (STWP) (1992) was developed using the target weight concept. The STWP was designed to be nonintrusive and clinically useful in long-term facilities with limited resources. It simply required the establishment of baseline and target weights and monitoring weights throughout the day.

The STWP was included as part of a comprehensive treatment protocol for disordered water balance. The treatment protocol entailed determining the baseline weight as an early morning weight prior to dressing, after voiding, and before any oral intake. The target weight was calculated to be 5% above the baseline weight. For example, a person weighing 150 lbs at 6 a.m. would have a target weight of 157.5 lbs. The target weight was established at 5% above the baseline weight rather than 7% recommended by Delva and Crammer (1988) because of the likelihood that the baseline weight was elevated due to urinary retention and interstitial edema. Individuals were weighed using the same counterbalance scale at regular intervals throughout the day (6 a.m., 11 a.m., 2 p.m., 4 p.m., 7 p.m., 9 p.m., 11 p.m.). These times were sometimes individualized depending on the client's activities. If the target weight was achieved, the person was prohibited from drinking any more fluids until the symptoms subsided. This usually meant that the person was restricted to the ward and ate meals on the unit.

This intervention differed from 24-hour seclusion recommended by Goldman and Luchins (1987). The goal was to prevent intoxication and re-establish normal fluid balance as quickly as possible with minimal environmental restrictions. Fluid intake was restricted, and the person maintained on "water observation." A person was to be in a staff member's sight at all times, observed for symptoms of water intoxication, and redirected from any fluid ingestion. Once the person's increasing weight gain was reversed and diuresis began, these restrictions were lifted. The restrictions were only to prevent water intoxication and were not viewed as consequences of over-ingestion of fluids. Typically, a client was restricted to a ward in the evening and ate meals without fluids.

In the mid-1990s, Leadbetter, Shutty, Higgins & Pavalonis (1994) developed a treatment plan that was comprehensive enough to detect acute hyponatremia. More specifically, the plan called for careful monitoring of body weight and periodically checking the serum sodium level. They used the client's diurnal body weight change to estimate the serum sodium level. A 5% gain in body weight, they estimated, was roughly equivalent to a 10 mEQ/L drop in serum sodium (Godleski et al. 1989). For example, if the client weighed 150 lbs in the morning and 157.5 lbs in the afternoon or evening (a 5% weight gain), the serum sodium level was estimated to be 130 mEq/L. This method assumed a normonatremic or "dry" weight in the morning When applying this formula, it was important to remember that it is the rapidity of change in the serum sodium level that presents the greatest risk to the resident (Koczapski and Millson, 1989).

By the year 2000, a great number of observational and speculative articles had been published about the etiology and treatment of psychogenic polydipsia and the relationship between psychosis and fluid dysregulation. The patients diagnosed with psychogenic polydipsia were typically managed with a combination of intravenous infusion of hypertonic saline, medications to oppose central vasopressin release, and diurnal weight measurements or target weight procedures (Vieweg, 1996; Koczapski, Ibraheem, & Paredes, 1985; Goldman & Luchins, 1987). The failure to find successful medical methods to treat this potentially lethal condition led to the use of behavioral methods to reduce liquid consumption. Promising results were reported in several case studies (e.g., McNally, Calamari, Hensen, & Kaliher, 1988; Pavalonis, Shutty, Hundley, Leadbetter, Vieweg, & Downs, 1992; Bowen, Glynn, Marshall, Jurth, & Hayden, 1990).

Thomas, Howe, Gaudet & Brantley (2001) utilized an outpatient behavioral approach in the treatment of psychogenic polydipsia with a nonpsychiatric, primary care, adult male client, suffering from intractable hiccup. The purpose of this case study was to illustrate a novel strategy for eliminating compulsive water drinking, thereby decreasing the likelihood of potentially fatal hyponatremia in a client refractory to traditional pharmacological treatments and behavioral interventions. The authors described the combined use of outpatient education, self-monitoring, medical feedback, behavioral reinforcement and reported successful cessation of polydipsia at 12-month follow-up. At eight-week outpatient behavioral intervention, the results indicated positive benefits in maintaining normal serum sodium concentration. Of Note: marked improvements were maintained when treatment was withdrawn, thereby dissuading the client and family from completing another course of treatment. Further, treatment gains were maintained for over 12 months. No attempts were made to involuntary restriction of fluid intake. The treatment techniques could thereby be applied in less restrictive settings, without the necessity of staff assistance to monitor and limit fluid intake.

Another outpatient case study (Costanzo, Antes, Christensen, 2004) suitable for higher functioning clients addressed several areas of behavioral change. Therapists used cognitive techniques to address thoughts leading to drinking behavior and then implemented a behavioral program to restrict water intake. They implemented a stimulus control paradigm that included positive reinforcement and coping skills. They followed the client with weekly visits for 12 weeks and addressed delusions and fears related to drinking excessively. The client used a record book for time, fluid amount, and situation for each beverage consumed. The client was given a 500 ml water jug as a stimulus control device and instructed to fill it only six times daily to achieve a goal of less than 3 L for water restriction. The client used coping skills (i.e., substituting ice cubes for drinks, taking small sips, distracting activities), positive feedback from the therapist and improvement of urinary frequency that reinforced fluid restriction.

SUMMARY

It is the author's opinion, which is shared by other professionals who work with clients diagnosed with psychogenic polydipsia (Cochrane, Goering, Durbin, Butterill, Dumas, Wasylenki, 2000), that tertiary residential programs may include community-based facilities. These programs provide transitional support for individuals moving from an inpatient setting to community residential facilities. They also provide ongoing support for individuals who have difficult-to-control behaviors, complex medical conditions, other serious deficits, and disabilities. In addition to having a cadre of highly trained staff involved in daily care delivery, community residential programs need backup access to inpatient services, respite care, and consultation/education. In conjunction, during the past 10 years, tertiary care models of support have been devised around portable, specialized, interdisciplinary outreach teams that serve the individual *in situ*. Their goals, among many, are to stabilize the situation, to avert hospitalization, to minimize length of stay in a more comprehensive tertiary setting (e.g., inpatient secured unit), and to allow the client when stabilized to return to the community residence.

Consultation is provided when the referring provider needs a higher level of expertise to manage a complex situation (Davidson, Cain, Sloane-Reeves, Giesow, Quijano, VanHeyningen, &

Shoham, 1995; Beasley, Kroll, & Sovner, 1992). Outreach teams are generally organized to provide urgent, but not crisis, response. To increase flexibility, the core staff of outreach programs can be supplemented with other specialists and contract workers from a range of disciplines as required (Cochrane et al. 2000).

Lastly, by the very nature of the symptomotology of psychogenic polydipsia, tertiary care is the most viable treatment approach with this clinical population, whether it be located in a secure hospital setting or in a community-based residential care centre. Behavioral indications of psychogenic polydipsia include: aggressiveness, noncompliance with medication, and danger to self and /or others. Most individuals diagnosed with this problem cannot be managed without higher levels of support provided by tertiary care programs. A primary theme throughout this book is that tertiary care does not necessarily require inpatient settings, provided appropriate community-based services are adequately staffed by professionals with an expertise in treating clients with this co-occurrent disorder.

CHAPTER TWO

A Comparison of Treatment Programs for Psychogenic Polydipsia

PUTTING INTERVENTIONS INTO PRACTICE

A variety of treatment programs developed for psychogenic polydipisa (1992-2006) has been chosen for perusal and in most cases are written verbatim from the extant article. Both inpatient and outpatient programs are included to provide different treatment interventions that have worked with varying degrees of success for this difficult and perplexing clinical population. The articles provide a "mix and match" of authentic challenges to combat the problem of psychogenic polydipsia. They should hopefully influence creative ways to enable the reader to develop residential treatment models in the community.

1. WESTERN STATE HOSPITAL TREATMENT PROCEDURE, STAUNTON, VIRGINIA (1992)

Pavalonis, Shutty, Hundley, Leadbetter, Vieweg & Downs (1992) chose a treatment approach for psychogenic polydipsia that included: behavioral intervention on an open psychiatric unit, which also addressed the threats to generalization that plagued earlier treatment approaches with inpatients attempting to live successfully in the community. Initially, this approach was developed based upon positive reinforcement, which included patient input and staff feedback about performance. This strategy conformed to patient rights while recognizing that the ultimate goal was for the patient to be discharged to a less restrictive setting. Pavalonis' team members promoted a more active role by the patient in their treatment through the selection of reinforcers and the development of self-monitoring skills. Finally, since continuous control of fluid intake was not deemed feasible or appropriate on the ward, they chose as dependent variables, indirect laboratory measures such as urine creatinine levels, and diurnal weight gain as estimates of fluid ingestion. Baseline data included weekly measures of diurnal weights, serum sodiums, serum osmolarities, urine creatinines, urine specific gravities, and urine osmolarities. Diurnal measures were taken for 23 consecutive weeks. This protocol involved daily monitoring of patient weight at 6 a.m. and 4 p.m. to detect rapid weight changes due to fluid retention. Changes in body weight had been shown to be a clinically useful way of predicting when a patient was prone to hyponatremia, such that a 5% increase in baseline body weight was roughly equivalent to a 10 mmol/L drop in serum sodium (Godleski, et al. 1989). When serum sodium was predicted to fall into the hyponatremic range, the patient received a laboratory assessment of serum sodium. Just prior to implementing the behavioral intervention, the patient's weight was charted every hour while awake for 1 week in order to identify drinking patterns. These data revealed that the patient gained most of his weight from excessive fluid intake between 6 a.m. and 9 a.m.; this was followed by a seven-hour period (9 a.m. to 4 p.m.) when the patient's weight was relatively stable. The patient then drank excessively between 4 p.m. and 7 p.m.

Treatment

Based on the one-week observations, it was decided that the patient would be reinforced if he gained no more than 3 lbs from 6 a.m. to noon and another 3 lbs from noon to 8 p.m. Increasing the amount of time the patient spent in structured activities was not considered an option as a way to keep the patient away from water due to a pattern of minimal compliance in attending more than the required two activities per day. The limit of 6 lbs (approximately 3% of baseline weight) was set for patients over the 14-hour period from 6 a.m. to 8 p.m. This 6 lbs limit allowed the patient to maintain estimated serum sodium levels within acceptable parameters (above 130 mmol/L).

The patient and staff identified both immediate and long-term reinforcers to be used if the patient met the goal of less than 6 lbs per day. When the patient gained less than 3 lbs during the allotted time interval, the patient received both a token and verbal praise from a staff member for not drinking excessive fluids. The staff reminded patients to control fluid intake so that they could earn additional tokens at the next weigh-in if they gained less than 3 lbs. They could receive two tokens per day, and if they received both tokens in a day, they were able to choose an additional reinforcer that evening. These additional reinforcers selected by the patient most often included peanut butter cups and sodas. When their total accumulation of tokens reached 60, they could trade them for a staff-supervised dinner at a restaurant away from hospital grounds. If patients exceeded the weight limit at any weigh-in time, the staff informed them that they had done so and therefore had not earned a token. They were also reminded about what they had to do to earn a token and at what time they were to be weighed.

The treatment was evaluated for 23 weeks to determine the efficacy of the behavioral intervention. No modifications of the program were made. The intervention was reevaluated 13 months later over a 12-week period.

Results

During baseline, the patient's mean weekly diurnal weight gain was 7.1 lbs, whereas normalized diurnal weight gain was 3.83%. In contrast, the patient's mean weekly diurnal weight gain during treatment dropped significantly to 4.1 lbs, whereas normalized diurnal weight gain was 2.05%. *Normalized diurnal weight gain is expressed as a percentage by subtracting the 6 a.m. weight from the 4 p.m. weight, multiplying the difference by 100, and dividing the result by the 6 a.m. weight.*

The overall fluid consumption significantly decreased from approximately 10 L per day during baseline to 4 L per day during treatment. There were no differences between follow-up and treatment measures of diurnal weight gain, serum sodium level, frequency of hyponatremic episodes and estimated fluid consumption, indicating that the patient continued to benefit from continued treatment one year later. The clinical significance of these findings were remarkable. The patient was able to decrease the frequency of having blood drawn by 25%, which was accompanied by a decrease in the frequency of pharmacological and physically restrictive interventions. With the decrease in fluid consumption came a decrease in occurrences of urinary incontinence. Consequently, the patient required less topical ointments for dermatological rashes resulting from urinary incontinence.

Discussion

This treatment paradigm for psychogenic polydipsia was developed to reduce excessive fluid intake using diurnal weight gain as the dependent measure. A criterion for diurnal weight gain was based on the baseline serum sodium and creatinine level for the patient's weight. Although daily fluid intake was never directly measured, the patient quickly reduced daily fluid intake (as measured by diurnal weight gain) thereby consistently meeting the weight criterion required for access to a reinforcement menu that he chose. In addition, the patient demonstrated marked decreases in laboratory values indicative of reduced fluid ingestion during the course of treatment.

The study used an A-B design with an extended follow-up (Hershen & Barlow, 1976). Although the design did not conclusively demonstrate that the intervention under study accounted for the observed effects, the reduction in collateral measures, such as serum sodium levels and frequency of laboratory assessment, across baseline and treatment, did offer support for treatment effectiveness. A withdrawal of treatment and return to baseline was considered too risky, given the seriousness of excessive fluid ingestion. Despite the methodological limitations of the study, the intervention appears to have substantially contributed a *significant* decrease in the patient's diurnal weight gain and the beneficial alterations in laboratory values.

2. THE ST. LOUIS STATE HOSPITAL TARGET WEIGHT TREATMENT PROCEDURE (STWP), ST. LOUIS, MISSOURI (1992)

Baier & Gaertner (1991) found that monitoring diurnal weight changes as a direct measure of fluid balance was promising in the prevention of water intoxication and maintenance of normal fluid balance. However, in some long-term care facilities, there were often impediments to implementing a simple intervention.

In this situation it was not possible to use serum concentrations to determine the actual hyponatremic state once a target weight was reached. Laboratory facilities were limited or nonexistent, and it was impossible to implement procedures requiring frequent "stat" laboratory results. Consequently, Boyd, Williams, Evenson, Eckert, Beaman & Carr (1992) developed an intervention that was effective, but also nonintrusive, useful on a long-term basis, cost effective, and easily implemented in other residential settings besides an acute hospital.

The St. Louis State Hospital Target Weight Procedure (STWP) was developed using the target weight concept. It did not have any intrusive procedures. *The STWP was developed to be nonintrusive and clinically useful in long-term care facilities with limited resources. It required the establishment of baseline and target weights and monitoring weights throughout the day. The STWP was to be included as part of a comprehensive treatment protocol for disordered water balance.

Treatment

The baseline weight was determined as an early-morning weight prior to dressing, after voiding, and before any oral intake. The target weight was calculated to be 5% of the baseline weight. The target weight was established at 5% because of the likelihood that the baseline weight was elevated due to urinary retention and interstitial edema. Individuals were weighed using the same counterbalance scale at regular intervals throughout the day (i.e., 6 a.m., 11 a.m., 2 p.m., 4 p.m., 7 p.m., 9 p.m., 11 p.m.). If the individual's target weight was reached, the person was prohibited from drinking any more fluids until the symptoms subsided. This usually meant that the person was restricted to the ward and ate meals on the unit. The goal was to prevent intoxication and re-establish normal fluid balance as quickly as possible with minimal environmental restriction.

The team chose to restrict fluid intake and maintain the person on "water observation." The patient had to be in a staff member's sight at all times, observed for symptoms of water intoxication, and redirected from any fluid ingestion. Once the person's increasing weight gain was reversed and diuresis began, these restrictions were lifted. The restrictions were only to prevent water intoxication and were not viewed as consequences of overingestion of fluids. A patient was subsequently restricted to the ward in the evening and ate meals without fluids.

To test whether or not a target weight procedure using only weights without serum samples was useful, a pretest/post test repeated measure design was used. For six weeks, urinary dilution and symptoms of water intoxication were monitored in subjects who were divided into two groups, with one group being assigned to the STWP during the last three weeks. Changes in urinary dilution and symptoms of water intoxication were compared between the two groups. It was recognized from the beginning that using urinary dilution and symptoms of water intoxication as dependent variables were not ideal.

To obtain an accurate assessment of the hyponatremic state, serum sodium concentrations should have been compared between the experimental and control groups before and after the intervention. This was impossible due to the lack of laboratory facilities, the intrusive nature of the procedure, and the unwillingness of the patients to have frequent venipunctures. The team decided that fluid balance/imbalance would be determined indirectly by two daily measures: urine specific gravities and the presence of symptoms commonly associated with water intoxication. These measures were determined Monday through Friday at 4 p.m. on the patients' units by the nursing staff trained in the procedures. Urine specific gravities were used as an indirect measure of fluid balance; because of the disordered water balance, patients had hypostenuria. It was reasoned that if the STWP was successful in restoring normal fluid balance, then urine specific gravities would approach normal. If the urine was dilute, then it was assumed that the vascular system had been overloaded. An instrument measuring the symptoms associated with water intoxication was developed for this study. The Water Intoxication Assessment Instrument (WIA) uses an 11-item scale based on symptoms of water intoxication, including restlessness, excitement, confusion, aggression, slurred speech, pressure of speech, tremors, edematous eyelids and face, distended abdomen, and hypothermia. Each item was rated from absent to severe on a five-point Likert scale. The intra-class correlation measuring inter-rater reliability was .67.

Results

The subjects were randomly assigned to the experimental (n=15) or control (n=15) groups. The mean age of the experimental group was 50 years (range 33-63 years), and 30 years (range 26-52 years) for the control group. Seven men and eight women were in the experimental group, and 10 men and five women were in the control group. Both groups were mostly European American: 13 in the experimental group and 11 in the control group. The other subjects were African American. The mean length of hospitalization was 13.5 years (range 1-30 years) for the experimental group and 12.5 for the control group (range 2-27 years). Most of the subjects were diagnosed with schizophrenia: 14 in the experimental group and 11 in the control group. Two persons in the control group were diagnosed with a bipolar illness, and the other subjects were diagnosed with atypical psychosis. Subjects in both groups had been diagnosed with a mental illness for more than 10 years. The mean number of years since diagnosis was 23.8 for the experimental group and 21.1 for the control group.

There was concern over whether the staff would regularly weigh the subjects because of frequent staffing shortages. Subjects were weighed at specified times and randomly observed by the researchers. However, during the fourth week (the first week for the STWP), there was some confusion on the part of the staff as to how the water restriction should be enforced. For example, could patients still go off the ward, or should they be restricted? On one of the wards, staff were not restricting the patients to the ward and there was no way of knowing whether additional fluids had been consumed. During week's 5 and 6, the last week of the procedure, fluid restrictions were strictly applied and were validated by the weight record.

The urine specific gravities (as measured on an ongoing basis) and the behavior and physical symptoms (as measured by the WIA) were monitored daily, Monday through Friday, between 4 p.m. and 5 p.m., the typical period for afternoon hyponatremia. Weekly mean scores of the

WIA and urine specific gravities of two groups were calculated and compared using MANOVA statistical techniques. The *experimental group's* specific gravities for the preintervention weeks (weeks 1-3) were 1.003, 1.004, and 1.004, respectively. During the intervention weeks (weeks 4-6), the specific gravities increased from 1.005 (weeks 4 and 5) to 1.007 during week 6. The experimental group's overall preintervention mean was 1.004 (SD = .002) and the overall specific gravity mean for the intervention weeks was 1.006 (SD = .003).

The *control group* did not experience a similar increase in the specific gravity measures. Prior to the intervention (weeks 1-3), the overall specific gravity mean was 1.008 (SD =.006); during the intervention weeks it was 1.007 (SD =.005). The control group's specific gravity means ranged from 1.008 in week 1 to 1.008, 1.007, 1.007, 1.006, and 1.007 in the following weeks. However, the standard deviations of the specific gravities in this group were quite large (.005-.007), indicating a broader range of specific gravity measures than in the other group. When the groups were compared before and after the intervention using MANOVA, there was a significant interaction between the groups and pre/post intervention. Thus, the use of the STWP for three weeks did increase the concentration of the urine, indicating that balance had improved. The WIA measurement of the two groups did not differ statistically or clinically. The mean scores in the experimental group ranged from 8.7 to 9.3 (weeks 1-3) and 7.2 to 8.3 in the intervention weeks (4-6). The overall experimental group mean was 9.1 preintervention and 9.8 during weeks 4-6. The control group was measured at a mean of 10.6 in week 1, to 7.6 in week 3, to 8.7 in week 6, with overall means of 9.0 preintervention and 9.3 during the intervention, weeks 4-6. It was interesting to note that both groups were elevated during week 5. This was interpreted by staff as a result of environmental influences, such as different staff members or new patients on the floor, rather than any changes in water imbalance. The WIA findings, although disappointing, may be related to the fact that many of the behavioral symptoms of water imbalance are also symptoms of psychosis or may be outcomes of water restriction, such as increasing restlessness.

Discussion

The use of the STWP as an intervention that prevents water intoxication was supported. The positives in urine specific gravities indicated that the individuals' urine dilution approached normal when using the STWP. It was also possible to successfully use this procedure on wards that are traditionally short-staffed. The WIA may be useful in determining how individual clients respond to an increase in fluid overload, but was *not* useful in preventing water intoxication. Because the symptoms of water intoxication are similar to psychoses, the data needed to be considered within the context of the clinical picture. Boyd et al. (1992) continued to include the STWP in the water intoxication/imbalance protocol with daily monitoring of afternoon urine specific gravities and symptoms of water intoxication. Including the use of the specific gravities and WIA as a part of the STWP helped the nursing staff interpret the significance of the weights. That is, if a client stayed within the target weight and the specific gravity and WIA was normal, it was assumed that the individual was staying reasonably balanced. If, however, a client was consistently below the target weight but the specific gravity was dilute, further investigation was indicated; either the baseline weight was wrong or the kidneys were unable to appropriately dilute the urine. For these patients, a serum sodium concentration was needed. If a client had a rapid increase in weight above target weight but the specific gravity was normal, the client could be ingesting fluid and had not yet excreted excessive fluid. In this case, the client was at high risk for water intoxication and a serum sodium concentration would be drawn. Fluid restriction would be implemented until further assessment was completed. If there was a gradual increase in weight over several days but the specific gravity remained normal, the individual may be increasing adiposity.

The study further detailed postexperimental results: four subjects were discharged from the hospital once their "water problem" was under control; two resided in boarding homes where the staff monitored their weight. In another example, once fluid balance was restored, the individual was instructed to self-monitor and lived in a group home.

3. LOGANSPORT STATE HOSPITAL TREATMENT PROGRAM, LOGANSPORT, INDIANA (1993)

Cosgray, Davidhizar, Giger & Kreisl (1993) developed a treatment program for patients diagnosed with psychogenic polydipsia that utilized control and monitoring, as well as psycho-educational approaches in one-to-one and group settings. In addition to individualized treatment strategies that were part of each patient's individual treatment plan, the patients participated in the treatment strategies that were part of the group program.

Treatment

Fluid restriction was the cornerstone in this treatment program and is a central strategy in the group program reported in this treatment approach. Nine patients were monitored continuously by a psychiatric attendant in a designated area of decreased stimuli by staff who had been trained to respond to patients with behavioral patterns manifesting water intoxication syndrome. One half of the area of a 25-bed closed psychiatric unit was used for the *controlled* therapeutic milieu for the treatment program.

As an environmental control variable, access to water was controlled (i.e., water fountains were turned off), rest room facilities were continually supervised, and meals were served on the unit with monitoring of intake by nursing staff. The need to control water was felt to be so paramount to successful treatment intervention that nursing personnel dispensed all fluids, including water. Each patient was allowed an allotment of fluids, including water that could not exceed 3,000 ml/day. Each patient's weight was monitored at least twice daily and a urine specific gravity was done once weekly on each patient. In addition, serum electrolytes and osmolality levels were done once weekly initially, and thereafter once every other week. A monitoring form was maintained on each patient on an ongoing basis. Initially, patients were totally confined to the unit, with all activities carried out on the unit. Gradually, the restrictions were relaxed to include: supervised half-hour sessions three times weekly to the canteen being allowed. After two months of restriction in the program, one patient who had been a member of the hospital basketball team was able to go on an overnight trip to a tournament at another state hospital and successfully self-limit fluid intake. A few weeks later, he was able to visit with parents off the ward, and he continued to self-limit.

This program utilized a psycho-educational approach to assist clients in assuming control over negative behavior manifesting the need for excessive water intake. Other dynamics of the psycho-educational approach included: providing opportunities for patients to discuss why fluid intake restrictions were needed, clarifying ideas about the necessity for fluid restriction, and providing explanation in behavioral terms of the consequences of water intoxication and the recognition of symptoms, such as increased irritability and demanding behavior. Psycho-education occurred both in one-to-one settings, with any member of the treatment team involved with patients on the unit—social worker, rehabilitation therapist, physician, nurse, psychologist and clinical nurse supervisor (CNS)—and in a regularly scheduled group, led by the CNS and a member of the psychology staff.

Another objective of the program was to assist patients in developing a sensitivity and awareness about negative behaviors that trigger excessive water intake in order to gain control of these behaviors. In a group setting, patients discussed methods of controlling excessive water intake such as chewing sugarless gum and talking with staff in response to the urge to drink water. Patients also discussed feelings about their inability to satisfy thirst on demand. There were also planned opportunities for discussion that allowed patients the freedom to develop plans to gain control of their own behavior. It was anticipated that some of the patients would be able to learn self-limiting behavior and would progress to care on units with less control and subsequently to discharge into the community.

Results

All patients' blood studies (i.e., serum electrolytes, serum osmolality, and urine specific gravity) were within normal ranges from the commencement of the program. The urine specific gravity, which had varied from 1.000 to 1.006 with a mean specific gravity of 1.015 for the nine patients, had increased to 1.022, with a mean gravity of 1.015. The mean weight of the respective patients at the program's implementation was 170 lbs; three months later, the mean weight was 160 lbs. Weights did not vary significantly from morning to night, although before the program variation occurred as much as 5-15 lbs. The use of posey belt restraints to control water drinking had decreased from a total of 1,303 hours for the nine patients in the three-month period preceding the program to a total of 20 hr 55 minutes in the three-month period after the program was implemented.

All patients experienced posey belt restraint before the program to prevent water ingestion. Restraint use on all patients decreased after the initiation of the program, with four patients having no restraint and three having 15 minutes of restraint or less. Two patients not on the program but on the same ward seemed to obtain vicarious benefit from the program, with a drop from 11 hr of restraint in the three months before the program, to "one use" after the onset of the program and 5 hr before the program, to "no use" after the onset of the program.

Behavior indicators demonstrated a lessening and stabilizing of escalating psychotic behavior since fluid intake was controlled. External water-monitoring control continued to be lifted to allow for increasing self-control by patients. Three times weekly, half-hour supervised trips to the canteen were added to the patients' activity schedules.

Discussion

At the time of implementation of the treatment program in 1993, the authors stated the patients reported increased self-esteem, reduced periods of anxiety associated with increased water drinking behavior, and an overall satisfaction gained from the ability to self-limit the amount of water consumed. The patients reported feeling physically better and identified decreased agitation and psychosis. A high level of staff satisfaction was associated with the program's apparent success in decreasing the problematic water-drinking behavior and the subsequent decrease in psychosis.

4. MOHAWK VALLEY PSYCHIATRIC CENTER TREATMENT PROCEDURE, UTICA, NEW YORK, (1997)

Visalli's (1997) article on developing a best practice model for care of patients with psychogenic polydipsia was initiated as a result of reviewing the then-current practice of care for this clinical population at Mohawk Valley Psychiatric Center. He found that a small group of patients required a large amount of one-to-one staff time for little or no long-term benefit. There was no uniform approach to identify, treat, and monitor outcomes for patients with polydipsia.

Treatment

When a patient was suspected of having psychogenic polydipsia, each of the assessments/protocols was initiated and completed. The initial goal was to gather baseline data and confirm or rule out the diagnosis. Clozapine is an atypical antipsychotic agent that has different properties from typical antipsychotic agents and has proven an important ingredient in the management of psychogenic polydipsia and persons with addiction problems. Concurrently, the dose and length of trial for the current medication was reviewed if the team was considering switching the patient to clozapine (the current medication may or may not have been clozapine). The team members, in conjunction with the patient, determined the course of treatment. If the patient was already on Clozapine, then the patient's response to the medication was evaluated and changes made accordingly. If the patient was not on Clozapine, the final determination to use Clozapine was made, if medically suitable.

Clozapine was monitored according to the original Clozapine protocol and clinical response was measured using a basic psychiatric rating scale at specific intervals. It was found that as the patient's condition improved, a positive psychiatric response and a major reduction in fluid consumption may or may not occur within the same time frame. Eventually there was an improvement in both areas.

Since many of the patients had a concurrent substance abuse problem, they were often involved in a mental illness chemical addiction group (MICA) as well as other psycho-educational and/ or smoking cessation groups. The goal was to have the patient gain insight and verbalize the benefits of positive behaviors such as abstaining from drugs and alcohol. The staff monitored the patient's level of participation in each of the preselected groups to measure whether treatments had been effective. Staff continued to provide feedback to team members concerning the patient's level of participation in the groups.

As patients responded positively to Clozapine, they become more amenable to group therapies. The Polydipsia Rating Scale (PRS) was designed to assess the patient's cognitive and physical status. This was important since weights alone may not have provided an accurate clinical picture of excessive fluid intake. In conjunction, some patients were bothered by the task of getting on the scale six times per day and had, in some cases, misunderstood the purpose of the weights and had responded by not eating. The rating scale was an additional tool used to help confirm a suspected polydipsia problem.

The weight protocol was initiated when the patient was suspected of excessive fluid consumption. The patient's weight was monitored on a weight table, and the difference between the morning and evening weight was not supposed to exceed 5% (Verghese, de Leon, & Simpson, 1993). When this occurred, the physician was notified because a rapid fluid shift may have produced marked changes in the patient's electrolytes, causing seizures. At some point, the patient was taught to monitor his or her weight. The number of daily weights were adjusted according to the patient's progress. This protocol then became part of the generic polydipsia behavior contract. Collaboration with a psychologist occurred at the time the weight chart was initiated. The monitoring process ensured the patient's safety while a more individualized behavior contract was being formulated.

A generic behavior contract was initiated when problematic polydipsia-like behaviors were suspected and/or identified. The use of tokens and other motivators was identified as useful behavior modification tools and was incorporated into the plan (Baier & Gaertner, et al., 1991; Bowen, Glynn, Marshall Kurth, & Hayden, 1990; Liberman & Marshall, 1993; Pavalonis, Shutty, Hundley, Leadbetter, Vieweg & Downs, 1992).

The contract provided rewards for positive behavior, such as limiting fluid intake, and was aimed at stabilizing the patient's weight. The plan was then modified for specific target weights and/or behaviors and was tapered according to the patient's response to treatment. It may have been terminated once the patient reached the desired outcome, or it may have been continued as reinforcement until the patient was discharged from the hospital.

Basic patient teaching was initiated by nursing staff to help patients examine the diagnosis of polydipsia, why people consume excessive amounts of fluids, and the relationship between excessive consumption of fluids and its consequences. Individual therapy was used to reinforce the information and assist the patient in striving toward his or her goal.

Family members were also involved in teaching. If the patient was not on Clozapine, and it was medically indicated, then the patient and his/her family would be given the opportunity to explore this treatment. Health teaching about the benefits of Clozapine was initiated. A video and/or other teaching materials was used to help the patient gain understanding of the benefits of Clozapine. Patients also found it helpful to meet with peers who had benefited from this medication. The goal of health teaching was to help the patient understand what treatment options were available and what to expect with each intervention. Once the information was provided, the patient chose whether or not to participate.

Results

The treatment team members collaborated to assess the results of the screening tools outlined and to establish an initial plan of care. The treatment plan reflected the choice of medications and other interventions for a specified length of time. The treatment plan and/or problem list reflected the patient's major deficits as a result of identified behaviors and a subsequent diagnosis of polydipsia. The list of problems and corresponding interventions were then prioritized. Setting priorities from a problem list helped treatment team members gain consensus in their approach to care. The plan was reassessed periodically.

As the patient progressed through the care map and was discharged from the treatment facility, the nursing discharge summary was initiated. It included health teaching components for polydipsia, which helped the next provider gain information about polydipsia and ensured continuity of care. Most discharged patients were familiar with this information and worked with the next provider to ensure these interventions continued in the community (i.e., generalization).

Discussion

The benefits of developing a care map (Visalli, 1997) included: increased interdisciplinary communication; better integration of the work of different disciplines on treatment teams faced with polydipsic patients; the development of the initial care map for polydipsia diagnosis and treatment; identifying a successful Clozapine trial as a major component in addressing a patient's psychosis and polydipsia; information for patient monitoring and discharge planning; diagnostic procedures subsequently based on observation and laboratory testing; the development of a generic weight monitoring program; the development of a generic behavioral contract; and the development of a flowchart of the diagnostic and treatment process.

The diagnostic procedures and care map were developed after a care team's retrospective study of three polydipsia patients on Clozapine was completed. The individuals were successfully treated and discharged to the community for one year. The care map represented an endeavour to define best practice guidelines for addressing psychogenic polydipsia and monitoring outcomes. This protocol was used for six months and led to a number of patients diagnosed with psychogenic polydipsia being discharged on Clozapine. None of the patients returned to the hospital, and all were doing well six months later (at the time the article was published in 1997).

5. MAYO CLINIC NICOTINE DEPENDENCE CENTER OUTPATIENT TREATMENT PROCEDURE, ROCHESTER, MINNESOTA (2001)

Thomas, Howe, Gaudet & Brantley (2001) described the treatment of psychogenic polydipsia with a non-institutionalized primary care patient with intractable hiccups. The article illustrated a novel strategy for eliminating compulsive water drinking, thereby decreasing the likelihood of potentially fatal hyponatremia in a patient refractory to traditional pharmacological treatments and behavioral interventions. The authors described the use of outpatient education, self-monitoring, medical feedback, and behavioral reinforcement and reported successful cessation of polydipsia at 12 month follow-up.

Treatment

An ABA single-case design was employed to evaluate the hypothesis that outpatient behavioral treatment targeting education regarding: intractable hiccups, behavioral reinforcement for decreased fluid consumption, and relaxation training would restore and maintain normal sodium concentration in a single, 48-year-old, unemployed, African-American male with a 21-year occupational history in landscape maintenance. He was referred by his treating physician for evaluation of compulsive water drinking, following elimination of all alternate medical causes of hyponatremia. At baseline, the patient was estimated to consume approximately 10L of water per day. Seizure activity related to his low sodium level was noted on two of his prior hospital admissions. The baseline phase (A1) was established using sodium concentration levels recorded during routine medical examinations, and hospitalizations over the prior four-year period.

During the eight-week treatment phase, the patient was seen for weekly 90-minute individual and family treatment sessions. These sessions were followed by visits with the primary care physician, during which time the patient was given feedback regarding his serum sodium level and referred for serum sodium levels. During treatment sessions 1 and 2, the patient and his family were provided education regarding the health consequences of excessive water consumption, including gastrointestinal distress, dizziness, malnutrition, bladder change, and central nervous system dysfunction. The educational component of treatment included a review of the health consequences associated with hyponatremia, and the patient was strongly encouraged to follow recommendations regarding regular use of chlorpromazine to manage hiccup episodes. During treatment session 2, the patient was instructed to use a four-ounce cup when drinking to increase awareness of the number of times he filled his glass. The patient was instructed to have no more than 64 ounces of liquid per day (16 four-ounce cups). An emphasis was placed on "all liquids," as the patient substituted apple juice and milk for water during the first week of treatment. Additionally, the patient was encouraged to self-monitor fluid consumption by recording each glass consumed on a daily fluid intake monitoring form.

During treatment sessions 3-5, the patient was taught alternate methods to cope with anxiety regarding intractable hiccups. He completed a reinforcement checklist that included possible items he would enjoy receiving as weekly rewards for normal sodium concentration levels. His family was encouraged to provide these items (e.g., baked goods) following weekly reports of normal sodium concentration levels. Positive activity planning was initiated during treatment session 6 as the patient's physical health began to improve (i.e., weight gain, increased strength, decreased GI distress, increased energy).

During session 7 and 8, problem-solving skills were taught to address difficult situations that arose during treatment (e.g., dehydration problems after spending time outdoors). Problem-solving training also involved generating a list of alternate behaviors for the patient to engage in when he experienced fear of hiccups and the resultant urge to drink excessive fluids. Such behaviors included distraction techniques (i.e., television, radio), physical activity, seeking social support and engaging in relaxation exercises. During each treatment session, overlearning was practiced by reviewing skills taught in prior sessions. Additionally, the patient received verbal praise from the therapist and physician during weekly sessions for satisfactory sodium concentration levels and progress reported by the family. The patient was also seen once per week, during which time medical feedback was given regarding sodium level. Approximately seven days passed between behavior (drinking), measurement (sodium level), and feedback. Serum sodium concentration was used as an indirect measure of liquid intake, as direct assessment was not possible in the outpatient setting. The target for treatment was a return of normal sodium concentration rather than a measurable reduction in fluid consumption. The patient's sodium level was assessed each week and progress was visually plotted and reviewed with the physician and family.

The final observation phase (A2) was established using sodium concentration levels recorded during 12 routine, monthly outpatient primary care examinations. Due to the stability of treatment effects and transportation concerns, the patient and his family declined an additional treatment phase (i.e., B2). The authors reported that it was not proven necessary.

Results

The mean serum sodium concentration for the baseline phase of treatment (A1) was 108 mmol/L (SD = 7.7; median = 106). The result of the baseline sodium range was communicated to the patient and family in visual form.

The first treatment phase (B1) began one week following hospital discharge. The overall mean level of serum sodium concentration during the treatment phase (B1) was 135.71 mmol/L (SD = 3.63; median = 135). The withdrawal of treatment phase (A2) was not characterized by a marked deterioration in overall serum sodium concentration (mean = 137.22 mmol/L, SD = 3.70; median = 136). Although a final treatment phase (B2) was planned, the patient and family declined participation as treatment benefits were sustained over the three-month assessment period. At the time of the article's publication, treatment effects had been maintained for over 12 months, during which time serum sodium concentration levels had been assessed by the patient's primary care provider during the monthly maintenance appointments. The patient most significantly had not suffered any episodes of acute hyponatremia during this period of time.

Discussion

The results indicated that an eight-week outpatient behavioral intervention had positive benefits in maintaining normal serum sodium concentration. Marked improvements were maintained when treatment was withdrawn, thereby dissuading the patient and family against completing another course of treatment. Further, treatment gains were maintained for over 12 months. It was tempting to make definitive conclusions based on the successful outcome of this intervention; however, given that a single case design was used, it is best to describe these results as promising. It is possible that other mechanisms may have been responsible for the treatment effect, given the complex interaction of physiological and psychological factors in polydipsia (Bremner & Regan, 1991).

The treatment method described shares many characteristics with traditional behavioral treatment for polydipsia; however, treatment was provided on an outpatient basis, and no attempts were made to involuntarily restrict fluid intake. More specifically, the techniques described could be applied in less restrictive settings, without the necessity of staff assistance to monitor and limit fluid intake. Further, these results strongly suggested that therapeutic measures such as education, medical feedback, and behavioral reinforcement should be instituted early when psychogenic polydipsia is indicated, in order to reduce hyponatremia from developing (Siegler, Tamres, Berlin, Allen-Taylor, & Strom, 1995). This study indicated that involuntary fluid restriction can be effective in highly structured inpatient settings; however, it is theoretically less feasible in outpatient clinical settings.

6. ALBERTA HOSPITAL TREATMENT PROGRAM, PONOKA, ALBERTA (2001)

Hasting's correspondence (October 4, 2001) to Riverview Psychiatric Hospital described the Ponoka SIWI Program and entailed the following information.

One of 2 long-term rehabilitation units at Alberta Hospital Ponoka is a 25-bed, integrated unit where care is provided to patients who have been institutionalized for an extensive period of time (i.e., 5-20 years). The majority of the patients on the unit have a diagnosis of schizophrenia and have been in hospital approximately 5-20 years. Of these individuals eight (both male and female) had a secondary diagnosis of psychogenic polydipisa. The patients were integrated with other patients on the unit and involved in all unit programs and activities. Water sources were accessible on the unit, including a water fountain and washrooms. In addition, these individuals went off the unit and attended the hospital cafeteria or the patient snack bar on a daily basis. The prime focus was to provide these individuals with a high quality of life and provide physical safety for their well-being, which may be jeopardized due to excessive fluid consumption.

Treatment

Prior to the commencement of a self-induced water intoxication program, each patient was assessed and weights taken on a daily basis to determine a baseline weight for the specific individual. Once the baseline was established, the program commenced and the patient was weighed four times per day. The time frames were upon arising in the morning, prior to lunch, supper, and bedtime. The unit physician could order that the specific gravity of the urine be monitored in accordance with the weight. If the patient's weight was over 2.5 kg above the baseline, weight privileges were suspended until three consecutive acceptable weights were achieved. "Acceptable" meaning less than 2.5 kg over baseline. If the patient's weight was 4.0 kg over baseline, the patient was placed in room restriction and observation level is changed to Q15 minutes. This continued for 12 hr. When this portion of the patient's care plan was instituted, the attending physician or the duty doctor was contacted, and an order obtained. This was the care plan that was followed for the patients on the SIWI Ward until 1999.

In 1999 a quality improvement project was developed and implemented, with changes to the treatment program. The patients were segregated from the other individuals on the unit. They were placed on constant observation, and care was provided in a large day room on the unit where water was not accessible. The specifics of the revised treatment plan for the psychogenic polydipsia program were changed to include the following protocol: Weights were taken five times per day and urine specific gravity twice daily. With the assistance of the physician and dietician, an approximate amount of fluid required was determined for each patient, ensuring adequate hydration during a 24-hour period. The patient could consume to the maximum amount, but not beyond. Blood and urine tests were done weekly, and the patients could go off the unit for recreation outings with the staff. The amount of fluid allowed was decreased by 100 ml per day until acceptable amounts were being consumed. Data were reviewed by the physician on a daily basis. Patients were assessed weekly by the physician for stages of severity of polydipsia as per a mental and physical assessment. Patients were maintained on q15 minute observation periods and were involved in activities on and off the unit including their vocational programs.

Results

The amount of fluids consumed was reduced; however, the amount of fluids consumed remained higher than the recommended amount. Urine specific gravity was more concentrated (1.011-1.029). Baseline body weights were reduced; however, the patients' appetites were improved. Patient teaching programs proved to be ineffective due to the chronic nature of the patients' mental illness. In conjunction, best practice guidelines utilized by other facilities were ineffective for the patient population being managed on the unit due to the chronicity of the psychogenic polydipsia. The St. Louis Modified Water Intoxication Assessment also proved to be ineffective due to the chronic nature of the patient's mental illness and severity of polydipsia.

Discussion

When the patients were in a controlled environment with staff supervision and involvement, their weights and urine specific gravity were maintained within normal range. Conversely, when the patients were independent in their access to the environment, their weights were elevated, urine specific gravity was altered, and their mental state deteriorated to varying degrees. The unit environment was not conducive to the independence of the patients (i.e., access to fluids was unlimited). If the unit had been modified to allow greater control of fluid restriction, as monitored by the nursing station controlling water taps, bathroom utilities, etc., this could have influenced different results regarding treatment efficacy. Nevertheless, the increased staffing costs to effectively manage this high maintenance treatment program was felt justified as the patients were perceived as having "increased quality of life."

7. SELF INDUCED WATER INTOXICATION (SIWI) TREATMENT PROGRAM, RIVERVIEW PSYCHIATRIC HOSPITAL, COQUITLAM, BC, CANADA (2001 – 2006)

Cullen, Hlagi, & Godin (2001) submitted a comprehensive paper to the hospital's senior administration, which entailed an extensive review of the "water ward" (SIWI Unit) which had commenced operation in January, 1984. The SIWI unit was abolished in 2006, due to hospital cutbacks and the patients being transferred to a community facility in Vancouver, which is still in operation (2012). The following information was taken verbatim from their report.

Treatment

Prior to 1984, the management of patients diagnosed with psychogenic polydipsia was difficult due to lack of resources, the patients' tenacious efforts to acquire fluids, staff's inability to restrict them from doing so, and a lack of understanding of this syndrome. During the period from 1984-1991, SIWI patients were co-located on one ward in order to manage these patients the ward was locked. Fluids were restricted except when supervised by staff. Meals, bathing and even toileting were supervised to monitor and discourage excessive intake of fluids. Weekly education was provided and grounds privileges were granted based on patients' overall psychiatric and SIWI presentations.

In 1991 the SIWI unit was extensively renovated to include a water control panel in the nursing station, which gave staff the ability to control the flow of water in the sinks and showers. The toilets were replaced with waterless sinks, and the renovation included a bathtub that could be emptied in seconds. This provided the patients with more privacy "and made staff supervision easier and less confrontational." Baths and showers continued to be monitored, but with a modified shower curtain. A protocol for managing fluid consumption was established, allowing a fixed acceptable weight gain (3.0 kg for females and 3.5 kg for males) and grounds privileges were contingent on these parameters. Patients were weighed at 7:30 a.m., 11:30 a.m., 3:30 p.m. and 7:30 p.m. Should a patient exceed these established weights, they were then placed on a fluid restriction protocol, and confined to the unit, as per the protocol, which was as follows:

Kilograms above A.M Baseline Weight

Weight Gain (Men) Weight Action (Level 1 = restricted to the unit)
3.5-4.0:   Level 1 privileges until wt. decreases to less than 3.0 kg above baseline wt.

4.0-4.9:   Level 1 privileges remainder of the day plus the next day

5.0-5.4:   Level 1 privileges remainder of the day plus 1.5 days

6.0-6.4:   Level 1 privileges remainder of the day plus 2.5 days

6.5+:   Level 1 privileges remainder of the day plus 3 days, and notify physician

Weight Gain (Women) Weight Action (Level 1 – restricted to the unit)
3.0-3.5:   Level 1 privileges until weight decreases to less than 2.5 kg
above baseline weight

3.5-4.4:   Level 1 privileges for remainder of the day plus next day

4.5-4.9:   Level 1 privileges for the remainder of the day plus 1.5 days

5.0-5.4:   Level 1 privileges for remainder of the day plus 2 days

5.5-5.9:   Level 1 privileges for remainder of the day plus 2.5 days

6.0+:   Level 1 privileges for remainder of the day plus 3-days, notify physician.

For both men and women:

Not off fluid restriction by Level 1: one more day 10:30 p.m. (wt. must be below 3 kg)

Fluid restrictions while on Level 1: Level 1 privileges an additional day privileges

Drinking urine or bath water: Level 1 privileges 24 hours

Fluids were restricted, and no extra coffee, tea, water, etc., was allowed. The patients could only have milk with their regular meals. This was to ensure that the patients were not continuing to drink, but instead, voiding the extra fluids. Weights were taken every hour, and the patient was not allowed to shower or bathe. If the patient showed severe signs of water intoxication (i.e., disorientation, confusion, falling, aggression) or reached a weight gain of 6.5 kg temperature, pulse, respiration and blood pressure were obtained and the physician notified immediately.

Psychogenic polydipsia ratings were determined as follows:
Severe – patient has had weekly fluid restrictions and SIWI symptoms have been present prior to fluid restrictions;

Moderate – patient has had an average of one fluid restriction per month. SIWI symptoms were present prior to fluid restrictions;

Mild – no fluid restrictions in past six months. No SIWI symptoms in the past six months.

Discussion

As a result of the literature review, a service delivery review, and a patient profile review, three treatment options were developed and are outlined below:

Option #1

The SIWI water ward would become a normalized environment where all patients have access to water. The SIWI patients (n =14) would be co-located on the unit with other patients who require a secure (i.e., locked) environment for their protection, SIWI would be managed as a subservice of this unit. The severe SIWI patients would remain on a secure unit as long as they were at risk. Continuing work would be done by the treatment team to move the mild and moderate SIWI patients to open units as their conditions improved and they demonstrated the ability to self-limit fluid intake. The SIWI multidisciplinary team would provide consulting services to other teams as required to support the SIWI patients on other units.

Pros

- Improved quality of life for mild and moderate SIWI patients who will have normal access to water and the opportunity to learn to control their own water-drinking behaviors.
- Improved quality of life for non-SIWI patients.
- The environment is normalized and in keeping with the philosophy of psychiatric rehabilitation.
- Improved bed utilization for SIWI and vulnerable patients.

Cons

- Costs attached to the unit renovations and family anxiety to proposed changes.
- Staff anxiety (i.e., concerns regarding increased aggression and management problems, keeping patients safe).
- The necessity for increased interventions with severe SIWI patients that may include increased use of PRN, constant attentions, territorial confinements and seclusions.

Option #2

This option highlighted the management of the severe SIWI patients (n = 5) being dispersed among three locked units in the psychiatric hospital.

Pros

- Alleviate the nursing load of having all five SIWI patients on one ward.
- Patients would have normal access to water.
- The number of seclusion rooms per locked unit would be adequate if needed for excessive water drinking behavior.
- Less emphasis on SIWI symptoms and more of a holistic approach to patients.

Cons

- Increased numbers of staff needed to be educated and supported regarding signs, symptoms, and treatment protocols for managing patients with SIWI.
- Increased potential of patient/staff confrontations, thereby causing an increased risk of injury to SIWI patients on nonintegrated "behavior stabilization units," which tend to be a more aggressive environment.
- Marked family concerns regarding the transfer of patients to more aggressive units.

Option #3

Moderate and severe SIWI patients would remain on the water ward. A structured, waterless environment would be maintained. If possible, enhanced services on the Water Ward would be provided for patients with moderate and severe SIWI symptoms. The bed count would be reduced on the unit and specialized care and treatment for patients provided with a diagnosis of SIWI only.

Pros

- Fewer interventions from staff.
- Decreased PRNs.

- Decreased constant attentions and decreased seclusions.
- Decreased risk of water intoxication for severe SIWI patients as their access to water would be completely controlled by the structure of the unit.

Cons
- An area in the hospital would have to be dedicated to meet the specialized needs of a small percentage of the patient population.
- Moderate SIWI patients would have limited access to water and have less opportunity to learn to control their own water drinking behaviors.
- There would be increased risk of unit contamination to patients and staff if no water was in the washroom sinks or toilets.
- This would be an "abnormal" environment, not in alignment with principles of psychiatric rehabilitation. More specifically, the interventions, including environmental controls, focus on the weaknesses rather than the strengths of each SIWI patient.
- The interventions would not facilitate the process of recovery.
- The services would not be provided in a normalized environment; it would not enable patients to develop to the fullest extent their capabilities.
- This option would create a "care-taking culture" rather than an environment where patients are encouraged to be responsible for their own recovery. The patients would also have decreased autonomy and the treatment would not be individualized.
- There would be reduced cost effectiveness to operate and staff a small unit for patients with severe SIWI.

The recommended option chosen by the multidisciplinary team was the implementation of Option #1, with the following goals in mind:

- Prevent intoxication and reestablish normal fluid balance as quickly as possible with minimal environmental restriction;
- Implement interventions that are effective, but also unintrusive, useful on a long-term basis, cost effective and easily implemented in other residential settings (i.e., open units and community facilities);
- In support of the philosophies of psychosocial rehabilitation and "harm reduction," the goal of the unit would be to assist patients in self-monitoring their daily fluid intake. This would facilitate each patient determining how to remain safe and symptom free while managing individual daily fluid intake.

OPTION # 1 - COMPREHENSIVE SERVICE DELIVERY PLAN

The goal of the Riverview Psychiatric Hospital's SIWI program in 2001 was to provide a comprehensive range of services that were evidence based. This would include the following factors of care provision:

Environmental Changes

All water would be returned to the unit. The waterless "airline" toilets would be replaced with ordinary toilets that could be flushed by the patients immediately after use. The current water-less urinals would be replaced with ordinary urinals. Water would be returned to the sinks to enable patients to wash their hands in the bathroom immediately after using the toilets. The bathtub would be replaced with an ordinary tub with a drain. The control panel in the nursing station that controls all water on the ward would be removed. The hand-washing sink located in the hallway outside the nursing station would be removed. The sub-acute room would be renovated to provide a second seclusion room. Bathroom doors would be equipped with locks to provide night staff the option of locking the bathroom if necessary.

Psycho-educational Approach

Psycho-education would include a series of group education sessions to the SIWI patients. These groups would be "nonconfrontational" and "open ended." They would be designed to increase awareness of self-induced water intoxication (SIWI) syndrome and management strategies. Issues of denial would be discussed and the physical problems resulting from excessive drinking described using visuals. Patients would be encouraged to monitor their feelings and behaviors. This is a crucial point, as a diagnosis of psychogenic polydipsia is viewed as an addictive behavior that is always present.

Behavioral Management Strategies

For patients who are noncooperative with water restrictions and psycho-educational programs, behavioral management strategies are potentially effective. Behavioral strategies would include the following:

Explanation of the SIWI syndrome, including risk factors, symptoms and reasons for fluid restriction. Clarifying each patient's individual reason for drinking fluids to help gain a better understanding of SIWI. Identifying individual factors that contributed to water seeking behaviors. Maintaining the therapeutic relationship to foster communication.

Providing an opportunity for patients to participate in decision-making to develop plans to control their behavior. Contracting with each patient a transfer of responsibility of drinking back to the patient, including specified daily fluid allowed. Using the formula 37 ml per kg of body weight.

Showing the amount allowed in cups and developing tools to help the patients calculate fluid intake. Providing education regarding the importance of decreasing the use of nicotine, alcohol, caffeine, street drugs. As anxiety increases the urge to drink, taking measures to decrease the level of anxiety by providing stimulating crafts, games, non-anxiety-provoking activities. Providing daily relaxation sessions and coping techniques, in conjunction with fostering a relaxed, quiet environment.

Allowing rest periods of 5-20 minutes throughout the day. Developing strategies to manage the urge to overdrink such as: delaying the urge through thought stopping, counting 1-8 while visualizing the numbers, diaphragmatic breathing to increase emotional control; drinking from a small cup; slowing down drinking time; drinking through a straw; eating hard candies rather than drinking; chewing gum.

Proposed SIWI Integrated Plan of Care

An integrated plan of care with a SIWI focus was suggested. The patients would self-limit their fluid intake and be free of harm due to SIWI symptoms. Nursing would develop a therapeutic relationship by maintaining a positive, nonjudgemental approach.

A baseline weight was taken in the AM (no shoes, coats, in day clothing) after the patient's first void. Baseline weight was only accurate if the patient had not been drinking during the night. Weighing each SIWI patient (4 times daily – QID) at 7:30 a.m., 11:30 a.m., 3:30 p.m., and 7:30 p.m.

When the weight was increased from baseline (literature suggests 5%) the patient was at risk and placed on fluid restriction. The duty doctor was informed regarding seizure precaution. Documentation included all signs and symptoms of SIWI, as well as changes in psychotic symptoms and paying attention to anxiety components.

Every shift was documented while the patient was on fluid restriction. When a patient was on fluid restriction no extra fluid was given to them. Meals were supervised and the SIWI patients were only to drink milk on their tray. The vital signs and blood pressure were monitored while the patient was on fluid restriction every shift or every hour when neurological symptoms were present.

When patients were on fluid restriction, they were to remain on the unit except for prescheduled structured activities; the patient had already signed a contract to avoid fluids. The patients remained on fluid restriction until their weight was within 5% of their baseline weight. Weights were completed every hour. While on fluid restriction, bathing was supervised. When on fluid restriction, charting was to be done each shift. If the weight gain was more than 6.5 kg or showed severe signs and symptoms of water intoxication (i.e., disorientation, confusion, falling), the patients were to be placed on special attention/constant attention for seizure precautions, vitals taken and the duty doctor contacted. "Stat" serum sodiums were likely to be ordered at this time. Patients' access to grounds and off-ward activities were contingent on their weight gain.

SERVICE DELIVERY PLAN—INTERDISCIPLINARY TEAM FUNCTIONS AND RESPONSIBILITIES

Psychiatry

The psychiatrist assisted and supported staff with patient education and transition. They were also involved in one-to-one counseling with each SIWI patient regarding new protocols. The psychiatrist completed a psychiatric assessment of each SIWI patient to determine optimum treatment. They reviewed medications (e.g., Clozapine) and administered the PANSS assessment regarding positive and negative symptom evaluation.

Physician/Medical

The physician monitored weekly electrolytes and urine for each SIWI patient, lab results, liver/renal and endocrine function, ADH. The physician completed a medical assessment of each SIWI patient to exclude any physical cause of SIWI, and to rule out all other medical conditions. A neurological exam was provided, including: CT scan; central positive myelinolysis; glucose tolerance to rule out diabetes; osteoperia and osteoprosis.

Occupational Therapy/ Recreation Therapy

These disciplines formulated a well-developed program with some joint programming with social work to enhance community preparation, offering a wide range of activities with input from patients. They provided regularly scheduled, highly structured activities both on and off the unit (i.e., games, exercises, daily relaxation sessions, leisure education and counseling). The disciplines assisted in psycho-educational groups for patients; teaching coping skills for dealing with water urges; teaching responsible drinking habits; enhancing choices and alternatives.

Dietician

The dietician assisted the team in developing calculated daily fluid requirements for each patient based on weight. This individual also assisted in developing a formula for maximum allowable weight gain within safe limits for each patient and monitoring dietary requirements. The dietician also developed a life skills program, assisted in the patient psycho-educational groups and provided various apparatus to enhance the seminars. In conjunction, the dietician provided dietary alternatives to drinking water such as gum, straws at fluid times to "slow down" drinking, and decaffeinated coffee to help decrease anxiety/agitation levels.

Social Worker

The social worker met with community partners to liaise on behalf of the SIWI residents regarding behavior, risks, and supports necessary to maintain the patients once discharged to the community. The social worker worked with partners in the community to increase visit and leave opportunities for patients. The social worker visited boarding homes to provide up-to-date knowledge and best practice information about SIWI syndrome, signs, symptoms, and behaviors. The social worker invited community partners from mental health teams, regions and boarding homes to unit rounds (i.e., meetings) to liaise and learn from the treatment team. The social worker participated in joint programming with the RT/OT regarding patient outings, community orientation and preparation. The social worker liaised with family members to provide reassurance and support during the patient's transition from the SIWI unit to open hospital units, with the goal of eventual discharge to the community.

Psychology

The psychologist provided general psychological assessments and for more extensive evaluation referrals to neuropsychological testing. Behavioral management plans were designed for each patient. More specifically, an array of positive reinforcers was developed for SIWI patients and behavioral contracts as required. The psychologist assisted nursing staff in the management of abusive behaviors and substance abuse counseling to patients as required. The psychologist trained the multidisciplinary team in behavioral management program techniques and provided one-to-one counseling for the SIWI patients on a prearranged basis. In conjunction, the psychologist was utilized in the psycho- educational semiweekly groups which ran continuously from 2002-2006.

Nursing

The nursing staff assessed patients for symptoms of SIWI, provided therapeutic interventions as needed, evaluated outcomes, and documented these processes daily. The nursing staff monitored weekly lab results, including urine specific gravity, serum electrolytes, and sodium levels. These interventions included one-to-one counseling with patients, facilitating group counseling, addressing physical concerns, and partnering with physicians, interdisciplinary team members and families. The nursing staff developed integrated plans of care using a positive approach in conjunction with team members for each patient. The primary nurse clinician and psychologist worked together on these issues, with input and contribution from the other members of the multidisciplinary team. Using a partnership approach and psychosocial rehabilitation philosophy (PSR), the patient was partnered in the development of an Individual Plan of Care (IPC). Family members and patients were invited to IPC rounds for their contribution and feedback. The nurse clinician provided education and support to the nursing staff.

Pharmacy

Pharmacy provided a pharmacological profile of each SIWI patient. Pharmacy facilitated psycho-educational groups regarding current SIWI medications.

Staff Transition Plan

Staff were involved in the planning of individual patient treatment protocols. Staff updates were provided weekly. Staff education (e.g., behavioral programming) was provided once gaps had been identified. Staff concerns were addressed in a timely manner. Staff was supported throughout the process. All Unions were updated regularly regarding changes. An orientation package was developed to assist in training new staff and on-call staff. In addition, interdisciplinary team members on the ward where the program occurred had ongoing education in the recognition of clinical signs of polydipsia and water intoxication.

Patient Transition Plan

Patients were informed of changes once decisions were finalized and recommendations approved. All SIWI patients were provided with individual explanations about the program and signed a consent form that was approved by the hospital's research/ethics committee. One-to-one counseling with individual patients and the primary nurse, as well as with the psychiatrist, was ongoing. Patients were involved in their individual treatment plans. They were invited to meet with the treatment team and have an opportunity to express their concerns, provide feedback, and have input. Patients who were to be relocated to open units in the hospital were allowed as much transition time as needed. Everything possible was done to ease the patient's anxiety and fear of leaving the SIWI unit. This was influenced with visits accompanied by staff to the new ward, "day guesting" opportunities, and the psychiatrist visiting the new unit to provide staff education about signs and symptoms of SIWI. Support and treatment strategies were put in place before the patient was transferred, including QID (4 times daily) weighings and weekly blood work. Patients were regularly updated at unit community meetings and group discussion was encouraged.

Family Transition Plan

Family members were supported and updated on SIWI planning by the nurse clinician, medical manager and physician of the SIWI unit. Family members were involved with the SIWI patient care plans and had input into decision making and planning activities. Family meetings were arranged by the social worker of the SIWI program.

8. SELF INDUCED WATER INTOXICATION (SIWI) PROGRAM: RESEARCH STUDY (UNPUBLISHED), RIVERVIEW PSYCHIATRIC HOSPITAL, CO-QUITLAM, BC, CANADA (2001)

A research study by the SIWI treatment team subsequent to the reorganization of the program commencing in 1999 (Multidisciplinary Treatment Team-SIWI program, Research Study Summary Report, June, 2001) was completed, with the following critique of the aforementioned treatment model.

The initial purpose of the study was to assess the patients residing on the SIWI Unit to determine whether it was necessary for the Hospital to maintain a Unit specifically designed for patients with SIWI. The research project was intended to identify how severe the SIWI problem was for each individual and whether these patients could be integrated into other units in an environment without the tight controls of a locked unit.

A secondary goal of the study was to assess the value of refractometer readings as a measure of patient risk, and to compare the relative merits of weight gain, refractometer readings (i.e., urine specific gravity), serum sodium measurement, and observable symptoms as indicators.

Two groups of patients were included in this study. Patients who were on the SIWI Unit but who did not have their fluid intake restricted during the course of the study were identified as the no fluid restriction (NFR) group. The remainder, whose fluid intake was restricted, were referred to as the fluid restricted (FR) group.

Method

Thirteen residents of the Self-Induced Water Intoxication Unit (SIWI) were monitored for this study. Eleven were males and two were females. Five of the patients were on fluid restriction from the start of the study. These five were not given the same assessments and were included mainly to assess the usefulness of the refractometer. Baseline weights for the *NFR group* ranged from 66.0-98.8 kg. The program's dietician then calculated fluid requirements for these patients. These were based on a rate of 3.3 ml per kg of body weight and ranged proportionally from 1980 to 2964 ml. of fluid per day.

Procedure

Measurements in the NFR group began November 14, 2000, and continued for 11 consecutive days with two exceptions, the sixth and the ninth days. Measurements were taken four times per day at 7:30 a.m., 11:30 a.m., 3:30 p.m., and 7:30 p.m. The *FR group* was assessed between January 15-22, 2001, for eight consecutive days. The measurements taken at these times were of weight and urine specific gravity (USG) as measured by a refractometer. Symptom severity was measured by the Modified St. Louis Water Intoxication Assessment (MSLWIA), which rated symptoms on seven dimensions (i.e., restlessness, excitability, confusion, slurred speech, pressure of speech, tremors, aggression) on a Likert scale from 0 to 5.

The ratings were used to place patients in one of four stages of severity. This scale was designed to be used twice per day for each patient following five minutes of observation. Ratings were made for NFR patients only. At the end of each day (7:30 p.m.), daily fluid intake was measured for the NFR group. Patients were aware that data was being recorded for a study during the assessment period, although QID weighings for these patients were already part of their daily routine. The data was analyzed using SPSS for Windows, Version 10.0.

Results

Weight: Weight gain was calculated by measuring the patients' weights at 7:30 a.m. and subtracting that figure from weights obtained at 11:30 a.m.; 3:30 p.m.; and 7:30 p.m. At each time period there were some patients who lost weight and some who had gained. The average weight gain was smallest at 11:30 a.m. and largest at 3:30 p.m., which showed gains as high as 5.7 kg (i.e., 12.5 lbs). At 7:30 p.m., changes in weights shifted slightly downward compared to the 3:30 p.m. levels. Overall, the average (mean) change was relatively stable, with patients staying well within their daily guidelines.

Fluid Intake: Estimated fluid intake at the start of the study was correlated with mean actual daily intake for NFR patients. Amounts ranged from 1,980-2,964 ml. All individuals consumed considerably more fluid than the recommended amount calculated by the dietician. There was initially little correlation between the baseline fluid requirement calculation and actual daily consumption. When one patient's data was removed, the remaining patients were found to consume an amount that was highly correlated with the required fluid calculation ($r2 = .62$, *p* less than .05). Despite this finding, actual amounts consumed ranged between 170% - 372% more than this value. The one patient who was removed had an initial calculation that was higher than the other patients, but a relative consumption that was lower.

Serum sodium levels: Sodium levels in normal individuals range from 135-145 mml/L. Sodium levels were randomly sampled in patients when refractometer readings were low in order to determine if they would be predictable from USG. Although sampling was limited, no consistent relationship was detected between sodium and USG.

Urine Specific Gravity (USG): USG levels should normally range between 1.010 and 1.025. It is generally expected that patients with SIWI will have lower levels due to the dilution of the urine as a result of water consumption. In the study, a refractometer was used to ensure the accuracy of USG readings. Measurements were taken each time a patient was weighed. Most notable among the results was that low USG levels were rare early in the morning but later in the day, 33% of the patients in the study were 1.003 or lower. This was the level defined in the "Nursing Care Plan" (November, 2000) where patients were placed on fluid restriction.

Modified St. Louis Water Intoxication Assessment (MSLWIA): Ratings of stages of water intoxication on this scale were meant to identify patients who had mild, moderate, moderately severe, and severe polydipsia. Stage 1, the mildest stage, has two levels – Ia and Ib. At the severe stage (Stage 1V) patients must be stopped from drinking. This scale provided an objective measure of patient symptoms that could be correlated with the weight gain, specific gravity, and sodium levels. Unfortunately, these calculations were not possible because almost all the ratings on this assessment were 1a, indicating only the mildest signs of water intoxication. Of a total of 157 ratings, only 3 were not 1a.

 Discussion: The study was undertaken to answer two questions:

1. Which of the patients diagnosed with SIWI could be managed on an open vs. secure unit to keep them safe from complications of their excessive fluid consumption?

2. Was the use of USG as measured by a refractometer a better indicator of impending risk from SIWI than measuring weight gain?

The SIWI patients (n = 13) were divided into two groups: *group one,* those that had a history of frequent fluid restrictions and therefore a high likelihood of suffering complications from their SIWI if allowed unrestricted access to fluids (FR); and *group two,* those patients that showed controlled psychogenic polydipsia housed on the SIWI Unit and could potentially be managed in a less restrictive environment (NFR). It was the second group that the clinical team were most interested in the answer to the first question. The first group was only included in the study to answer the second question. The study design did prejudge the outcome of the first group.

More specifically, the team's clinical experience with this group over many years caused a reluctance to expose the patients to significant risk, validating a finding of which there was already a consensus; that the management of this group could not safely be provided in a less secure environment.

The patients in group two—the NFR group—were allowed unrestricted access to fluids until they reached Stage 111 of the Stages of Severity of the MSLWIA polydipsia scale. Other than one patient on one reading, all patients in this group did not score above Stage 1, demonstrating that they were able to control their fluid intake to a degree that did not make them symptomatic, despite unlimited access to fluids. While for many of the patients this result was not unexpected, the overwhelming absence of symptoms could be suggestive of several factors:

1. The patients were aware of the study and thus the closer monitoring had them controlling their fluid intake with greater scrutiny for the period of time they were observed;

2. The MSLWIA was a tool unfamiliar to the staff and this effected its consistent application, and;

3. The MSLWIA and how it was applied was not sensitive or specific enough to determine subtle changes in Riverview's SIWI population.

Despite these shortcomings, the clinical team felt that the trial adequately allowed a determination that *all but one of the SIWI patients under investigation could be tried on an "open" hospital unit.* One of the SIWI patients whom the team felt required a secure setting ingested the largest amounts of fluid in the shortest time frames (i.e., both high risk factors for symptoms) but balanced this by taking extra salt (noted after the fact by patient's own admission) in an effort to avoid having signs/symptoms of SIWI.

The patients were documented as consuming a considerable amount more than their calculated daily requirement based on their weight. This implies that their ability to avoid significant symptoms did not rely only on reducing their fluid intake but also on more efficient elimination. The figures for USG confirmed this, as the mean of USG's for this group of patients was well below population norms, indicating the patients excreted more dilute urine.

A commonly accepted threshold for intervention is a USG of 1.005. The findings indicated that this number was the mean for the Riverview SIWI patient population for the majority of a 24-hour day, and over a third of the SIWI patients had USG's at or less than 1.003, all without showing signs or symptoms of water intoxication based on the MSLWIA. It therefore appears that USG was not a good indicator of pending complications from excessive fluid intake in the Riverview population of patients with longstanding SIWI. Since USG's require an expensive instrument (i.e., refractometer) to measure and require the handling of urine, the practical applications for this monitoring technique was also limited, especially for patients who were to be discharged from hospital.

The question remained—what monitoring technique was the most effective in predicting those SIWI patients who are at risk for complications? The lack of sufficient serum sodium measurements obtained during the trials precluded a definitive answer for this indicator. The results that were obtained lacked any clear relationship with weights or USG's. While a more formal study was required to answer this question properly, it appeared that none of the indicators examined were significantly better at predicting impending risk than weighing the patient against baseline, the technique the Riverview Hospital SIWI unit had been using for over a decade. In addition, weighing was the most practical technique for patients who were moved to other units or discharged and was the only technique that patients could use themselves.

With the large range in baseline weights and fluid consumption of the patients tested, it was clear that the single thresholds for weight gain for males and females was not appropriate. Individual thresholds established on the basis of an assessment of unrestricted fluid consumption (until the patient showed symptoms) minus their baseline fluid requirement and a reasonable safety margin (e.g., 25%) would give a safe volume a patient could consume in a day. This could then be translated into an allowable safe weight gain (i.e., 1 L of water = 1 kg) for that patient. The use of individualized thresholds was also more consistent with a psychosocial rehabilitation approach by replacing the institutional "one size fits all" model with an opportunity to custom-fit the treatment for each patient's specific circumstances. This would encourage more patient involvement and understanding of the illness and treatment needs.

9. EAST LAWN BUILDING – PSYCHOGENIC POLYDIPSIA "WATER WARD" (2002 – 2003) ANNUAL REPORT, RIVERVIEW PSYCHIATRIC HOSPITAL, COQUITLAM, BC (2003)

Planning For Change – SIWI "Water Ward" (2002-2003)

Upon commencement of employment at Riverview Psychiatric Hospital in December, 2001, the author was requested to "re-engineer" the current SIWI treatment paradigm that was in practice on the locked water ward. The directive was in harmony with the recommendations (see 7 & 8 above) made by the program's clinical practitioners in the spring and summer of 2001.

After reviewing the various documentation and recommendations for change in the treatment protocol, the author invested the better part of five years implementing the following changes. The subsequent information is a synopsis of the changes made until the termination of the Riverview SIWI program in 2006 due to British Columbia government cutbacks and policy revisions (i.e., discharging all SIWI patients to a community residential setting).

SIWI Water Ward – Modifications made 2002 – 2003

Three processes were used by the author to "re-engineer" the SIWI treatment program that was currently in practice upon his arrival in late 2001.

1. Create a vision and mission statement of the 12 SIWI patients receiving treatment on the water ward. Primarily, medical intervention regarding Clozapine as the medication of choice; behavioral modification procedures to reduce the tendency to overdrink and reinforce more appropriate drinking habits; and psychosocial rehabilitation in the form of psycho-education semiweekly closed, group meetings. Five modules were developed, including two taught by Dietary Services, two modules taught by Nursing and the final module being taught by Psychology.

2. Develop the staff's core competencies in behavioral management (i.e., behavior modification) its philosophy and practical application. A comprehensive daily, weekly, and monthly reward and evaluation procedure was adapted for the unit to carefully "track" the behavior of the respective SIWI patients. In addition, a formalized, ongoing quarterly review was established to provide a regular, team-focused critique of the day-to-day treatment of the patients monitored; and,

3. Develop the unit's guiding principles and implementation strategies regarding behavioral management, this approach being interfaced with a semiweekly, psycho-educa-

tional (PSR) closed, group program for which mandatory attendance of the SIWI patients was required.

In November 2001, an evaluation of the SIWI unit included a section of the report entitled "Re-development Proposal—Critical Path" which recommended the development of a formalized, psycho-educational teaching package (to commence in March, 2002) and the recommendation of a behavioral contract format to be developed by the SIWI Unit Psychologist and the Unit's Nurse Clinician (to be completed in January 2002). In December 2001 the author commenced employment at Riverview Hospital with an established background in developing/training/ evaluating behavioral management programs with various clinical populations.

In February 2002 the author met with the Vice President of Medical Services of Riverview and discussed at length the behavioral management and psycho-educational (PSR) training programs for the SIWI Unit; and the development/training/implementation/evaluation of the treatment program. From February to April 2002, the author developed a behavioral management training Module (I-VI) at a Community (Junior) College level of complexity (see Bernstein, Ziarnik, Rudrud & Czajkowski, 1981). The recipients of this training program were current SIWI nursing staff and health care workers; allied health care professional staff, including vocational; recreation; social work; occupational therapy; physiotherapy; pharmacy; physicians; and management who interfaced with the treatment of SIWI patients on the water ward.

The commencement of the SIWI Behavioral Management Training Module (I-VI) began in early April and ended in late May 2002. A pretraining Behavior Management Knowledge Quiz was completed and subsequently the same test given posttraining. The implementation of the behavioral management program on the water ward began (baseline training) July 30 for a pre-authorized time period of one month, ending August 30, 2002. Prior to this period, the author and the manager of the SIWI Unit met to discuss the behavior management program with the 12 SIWI patients' family members and answer any/all questions and concerns.

The feedback was generally positive, indicating that the introduction of this program could im-prove (i.e., potentially reduce compulsive fluid seeking behavior) the patients' internal control of seeking out and overdrinking any/all fluids and consequently improve their quality of life. During this period all patients of the SIWI Unit were debriefed regarding the nature of the behavioral management program commencing July 30 and more specifically for the 12 SIWI patients. No one "opted out" of the impending behavioral management protocol, in fact all the patients looked forward to the commencement of the trial period.

Baseline Results
The baseline (30 day) trial of the behavioral management program ended with the follow-ing results: The mild/moderate SIWI patients (n = 5) did not differ markedly regarding the number of fluid restrictions prebaseline and postbaseline. The severe SIWI patients (n = 7) increased their fluid consumption during the month of August. A cursory analysis of the test data indicated the mild/moderate SIWI patients remained the same regarding the tendency to

overdrink (i.e., necessitating imposed fluid restrictions) due to excessive weight increases and the severely afflicted SIWI patients' rate of fluid intoxication rose generally across the board. The psycho-educational semiweekly closed, group (i.e., SIWI patients only) was initiated in late August 2002 to complement the behavioral management program. The first draft of a six-module treatment design developed by the nurse clinician emphasized an educational orientation towards the SIWI patients gaining greater knowledge of SIWI and methods of reducing their propensity to overdrink fluids. Subsequently, the draft was revised (i.e., streamlined) and implemented in January, 2003 as a five module semiweekly (i.e., Tuesday, Thursday) closed, group process. This revised treatment design utilized the "dietary" discipline for two of the five modules. The second draft, by April, 2003 was well received by the patients and the SIWI Unit staff. As a result of the baseline trial which included: (a) test results utilizing the behavioral management program designed and implemented with the SIWI multi-disciplinary team trained in behavioral modification techniques; (b) feedback from the SIWI staff regarding the strengths and needs of the tandem programs (i.e., behavioral management; psycho-education); (c) extensive review of other SIWI programs in North America; (d) reviewing previous behavioral management programs on the Riverview SIWI Unit; a vision and mission statement of the behavioral management and psycho-educational program was developed.

Planning Effectively To Develop A Vision

The SIWI patients completed a baseline study (i.e., July 30-August 30, 2002) to test the behavioral management treatment feasibility with this clinical population. The multidisciplinary treatment team trained in behavioral modification procedures incorporating measurable outcomes, agreed that utilizing reinforcement strategies (i.e., daily, weekly, monthly) on a personalized basis with each respective SIWI patient would be an effective means of potentially increasing the patients' self-control regarding fluid consumption. In conjunction, commencing August 20, 2002, a semiweekly psycho-educational closed, group meeting for SIWI patients only, would also incorporate a cognitive-behavioral model of therapy (e.g., challenging automatic thoughts) regarding excessive fluid consumption.

Hoshin Planning

Kenyon (1997) states Hoshin planning is a combination of strategic planning and policy deployment throughout a unit, department, organization. The key elements of Hoshin planning, as applied to this program, are: (a) a planning and implementation process that is continuously improved throughout the year, a quarterly review of the behavioral management program, a semiannual review of the psycho-educational treatment groups; (b) focusing on key systems that need to be improved to achieve strategic objectives (e.g., examining the treatment delivery on a daily, weekly and monthly basis); (c) participation/coordination by all levels of the unit in the planning/implementation of the SIWI treatment objectives (e.g., increased self-control regarding fluid consumption); (d) planning/executing change based on facts (e.g., reviewing the data collected on a weekly basis); (e) goals/action plans regarding change in treatment delivery based on realistic staffing capabilities (e.g., ongoing examination of the staff capabilities/resources to carry out treatment objectives).

Based on the Hoshin Planning Model the following vision and mission statement was developed for the SIWI unit.

VISION

SIWI patients will increase self-control of fluid consumption to allow discharge from a locked hospital unit.

MISSION STATEMENT

1. The SIWI multidisciplinary team will utilize a combined therapeutic approach with the SIWI patients on the Unit. More specifically, utilize behavioral management principles to encourage increased self-control of fluid consumption by the patients. In conjunction, utilize semiweekly psycho-educational group meetings aimed at increasing knowledge about self-induced water intoxication and introducing simple, yet practical cognitive-behavioral techniques to challenge maladaptive thinking strategies and the propensity to seek out and overdrink fluids;

2. Extensive review of the literature indicated that a combined approach of pharmacological intervention/behavior modification/psycho-educational group therapy was the most effective methodology in reducing the need for excessive fluid consumption;

3. The multidisciplinary SIWI team treat patients diagnosed with psychogenic polydipsia, of which the majority suffer from the effects of hyponatremia (i.e., severe hyponatremia causes neurological and psychiatric symptoms referred to as water intoxication). The prevalence of Riverview Hospital inpatients suffering from psychogenic polydipsia and hyponatremia due to chronic and excessive fluid consumption is unknown. Of particular concern is evidence that chronic hyponatremia is associated with high mortality among SIWI patients. The SIWI staff have been trained to provide daily, weekly, and monthly reinforcers (i.e., personalized rewards) to the respective SIWI patients for appropriate fluid consumption. Each SIWI patient is weighed at 0730; 1130; 1530; 1930 hours and provided a fluid restriction if over a preset weight limit (i.e., 4 kg males; 3.5 kg females). Daily monitoring of the patients' respective medication regimen is carefully assessed as an important adjunct to the overall therapeutic interventions.

Principles of the SIWI Program at Riverview Psychiatric Hospital

Ideally, a successful treatment program of identified expectations is articulated entailing the following paradigm: (a) the treatment expectations are carefully explained to the patients; (b) consequently a series of behaviors are set in motion by the patient to acquire a reward; (c) a causal process is learned by the patient; (d) a desired effect occurs, such as a reduction of fluid overconsumption.

Due to the nature of the psychogenic polydipsia syndrome and the risk factors of open access to fluid resources, there was an ethical dilemma in utilizing a treatment design that included removing a treatment protocol to measure its effect on the SIWI patient's level of function. Consequently, the treatment approach at Riverview's SIWI "water ward" was duty bound to utilize a one-group pretest/posttest design from which a conclusion could not be made that those changes (e.g., reduction in overconsumption of fluids) were produced by the program as a direct cause-effect consequence. This "competing hypothesis" dilemma, asserts that although there might have been changes, other factors outside the program may have produced the changes.

Lastly, the usefulness of the SIWI data received on an ongoing basis provided current information from which to base decisions about patient treatment status vis-à-vis discharge to a less restrictive environment. In conjunction, the information generated was helpful in the control, planning and accountability of such a treatment approach allowing quantification of outcome measures from an effectiveness-based system.

Practice – Contributions to Treatment of SIWI by Unit Disciplines

Medicine:
- **Assessment:** Identify acute and chronic medical complications. Perform differential diagnosis.
- **Monitoring:** Oversee weight and serum sodium monitoring. Ensure comprehensive treatment planning.
- **Intervention:** Treat hyponatremia and medical sequelae. Manage pharmacologic intervention. Ensure implementation of psychosocial intervention.

Nursing:
- **Assessment:** Evaluate self-care abilities and deficits.
- **Monitoring:** Implement weight protocol. Identify needed adjustment to privileges and treatment plans.
- **Intervention:** Restrict fluid access. Administer treatment for hyponatremia and sequelae.

Psychology:
- **Assessment:** Evaluate neuropsychological, behavioral, and personality functioning.
- **Monitoring:** Observe patterns of fluid consumption. Identify psychological and behavioral changes.
- **Intervention:** Develop individual, group and unit-wide psychological and behavioral interventions.

Social Work/Vocational/Recreation Therapy/ Occupational Therapy
- **Assessment:** Evaluate psychosocial functioning and environmental determinants.
- **Monitoring:** Ensure realistic strategies are transferable to less restrictive settings (team consultation).
- **Intervention:** Plan discharge. Coordinate resources and services. Educate community care providers about SIWI patients.

Four Domain Self-Care Model (2002-2006)

The Riverview SIWI Unit followed a four-domain self-care model that included: (a) air, food, and fluid; (b) hygiene and elimination; (c) activity and rest; and (d) solitude and social interaction.

Patients with psychogenic polydipsia have alterations in each domain. In the air, food and fluid domain, any/all fluid loading may result in increased blood pressure or pulse, shortness of breath, edema, or abdominal distention. In the hygiene and elimination domain, skin integrity may suffer if the SIWI patient is incontinent. Patients can develop "hypotonic bladder" and have residual volumes of up to 1 L of urine. In the activity and rest domain, the patient may be suspected of being hyponatremic when the patient has afternoon exacerbation of the underlying psychiatric symptoms. Other signs of hyponatremia include restlessness, confusion, agitation, aggressiveness, and pacing. In the solitude and social interaction domain, patients isolate themselves to hide their drinking. Preventing such behavior requires frequent redirection and active observation by the unit's multidisciplinary team in addition to their regular duties with the other patients on the Unit.

Treatment Implementation of Revised SIWI Program at Riverview

The development/training/implementation/evaluation of the behavioral management and psycho-educational treatment protocols during the revision of the SIWI program (2002-2003) was both creative and challenging. The following information is a progression of treatment initiatives taken by the SIWI multidisciplinary team:

- From July 30, 2002, to August 30, 2002, the SIWI patients were weighed 4 times per day (7:30 a.m., 11 a.m., 3 p.m., and 7 p.m.) as a baseline practice run prior to initiating rewards (August 31) (see below). Each reward progressed in status hierarchy on a daily, weekly and monthly basis with predetermined personalized reinforcers (reward) for each SIWI patient for not overdrinking fluids (i.e., 4 kg for males; 3.5 kg for females). In addition, three criteria were assessed at each of the four testing periods: white poker chip (1 point) for punctuality at each weighing period; blue chip (2 points) for weight; red poker chip (3 points) for appropriate behavior since the previous weigh-in. Total potential daily points for not overconsuming fluids was 24, of which, 20+ points must be obtained to receive a personalized reward; weekly potential points (168) of which greater than 135 must be obtained to receive a personalized reward (of greater worth); and lastly, monthly potential points (672) of which greater than 525 must be obtained to receive a personalized reward, of greater worth. As an addendum regarding choice of rewards per respective patient, the literature on behavior modification methodology suggested that generalized rewards (i.e., the same reward for everyone) reduced the potential power of the reinforcement paradigm because of the idiosyncratic nature of people's likes/dislikes regarding rewards and their consequent power.

- Commencing August 20, 2002. the psycho-education semiweekly groups (i.e., six rotated training modules) were initiated Tuesday and Thursday mornings (8:30 a.m.- 9 a.m.) as an adjunct to the behavioral management program; attendance and punctuality were made mandatory.

- It was decided by the SIWI multidisciplinary team to formally review the behavioral management program every three months subsequent to its starting date (i.e., August 31, 2002). As well, it was decided to review the psycho-educational training modules in late fall-early winter 2002-2003. In conjunction, rigorous attention to the SIWI patient's access off unit was coordinated with their respective weight protocols and subsequent fluid restrictions for being over the proscribed weight criteria established for males (i.e., 4 kg) and females (3.5 kg). Thus, access to earning level 3 unescorted grounds meant compliance by the SIWI patient regarding the weight criteria. A unit restriction because of noncompliance would mean loss of access off unit. Obviously, the fluid restriction statistics kept on each patient would be affected by unit restriction. In conjunction, level 2 access, which requires staff-supervised grounds, would also reduce a patient's potential for overdrinking fluids. These treatment protocols had mediating effects on teasing out the effectiveness of the behavioral management program. During this period the SIWI staff controlled the water access to the SIWI patients from within the nursing station (turning on water six times per day, allowing a maximum of two cups of water per patient per scheduled time) in addition to the mealtime access to fluids.

- On October 10, 2002, the SIWI multidisciplinary team met to review the behavioral management treatment protocol and the following recommended changes were incorporated: the point score for weight was reversed with behavior consequently the color of the weight chip was changed to red and the behavior chip to blue. The staff felt that weight was a higher prioritized criteria in the treatment paradigm; if at any time the SIWI patient was placed on fluid restriction the patient would not be eligible for a daily reward; the topic of verbal praise was reiterated pertaining to daily, weekly, and monthly rewards (i.e., personalizing each patient's success when they achieved daily, weekly and monthly rewards for appropriate fluid consumption); the weekly data sheets were to be completed Monday night by the night staff and left for the author to review.

A change in the weight criteria was increased from 4 kg to 5 kg for males and 3.5 kg to 4.5 kg for females effective November 30 2002, as an attempt to tease out each SIWI patient's SIWI symptom threshold. These individuals had, over the years, become very adept at masking their SIWI symptoms when intoxicated. This procedure was abolished after one month and the former weight criteria reestablished (i.e., 4 kg for males; 3.5 kg for females).

- Commencing October 30, 2002, the controlled water access procedure was terminated and the water left on 5 minutes 3 times per day (i.e., 9:30 a.m., 1:30 p.m., and 5:30 p.m.). Simultaneously, juice and coffee were made available to the patients in an attempt to "normalize" drinking behavior by providing a choice of fluids for ingestion.

- In December 2002, the multidisciplinary team commenced a revision of the psycho-education training program, which was completed and implemented in late January 2003. The changes consisted of five modules instead of six; two modules being taught by Dietary Services; two modules taught by Nursing and the remaining module taught by Psychology.

- On January 27, 2003, the behavior management program received a second, formal appraisal by the SIWI multidisciplinary team with the following changes: (a) one choice of fluid (e.g., juice, coffee or water) at the daily fluid periods; (b) if a SIWI patient had a fluid restriction (FR) during the day they lost their daily point total regardless of previous points earned that day; and if a SIWI patient had two fluid restrictions in a week they lost their weekly point total and were not eligible for the weekly prize.

- On March 24, 2003, the availability of water from the faucet was increased from 5 to 15 minutes, three times per day, to be assessed in three months by the SIWI multidisciplinary team. Further discussion by the team was held in early April 2003 regarding future water availability and the mechanics of incremental increases (e.g., how much increase and in what time periods) vis-à-vis behavior management protocol.

As a result of staff discussions the author suggested the following time periods:
1. March-May 2003: 15 minutes "open water" (to be reviewed at the end of May) if successful; increase the duration of patient access to open water;

2. May-July 2003: 30 minutes open water (to be reviewed at the end of July) if successful; increase the duration of patient access to open water;

3. July-September 2003: 60 minutes open water (to be reviewed at the end of September) if successful; increase the duration of patient access to open water;

4. September-December 2003: 90 minutes open water (to be reviewed at the end of December) if successful; increase the duration of patient access to open water;

5. December-March 2004: 120 minutes open water (to be reviewed at the end of March) if successful; increase the duration of patient access to open water.

The analysis of the access to the water fountains (open water) was achieved with some success. More specifically, the patients with mild/moderate SIWI were able to engage in increasingly responsible fluid ingestion to 60 minutes of open water access. Beyond this time period (i.e., 90+ minutes) there was an increased tendency to relapse due to irresponsible drinking patterns emerging. The severe SIWI patients (n = 5) were unable to stop the urge to overdrink and had to be closely monitored by the Unit staff throughout the day and evening.

Overall, it appeared the "critical mass" for the duration of open water period was approximately 60 minutes for mild/moderate patients diagnosed with psychogenic polydipsia. There was no indication throughout the trial period that patients diagnosed with severe psychogenic polydipsia had the emotional control to ingest "open access" fluids without relapsing/decompensating.

Recommendations
From 2002 to 2006 the Riverview Hospital, multidisciplinary SIWI team treated 12 SIWI pa-

tients diagnosed with psychogenic polydipsia (i.e., mild to severe) from a biopsychosocial perspective (i.e., pharmacological, psychosocial and behavioral management). From this experience the following six recommendations were developed:

1. By April 2003 the three cohorts of the 12 SIWI patients diagnosed with mild, moderate, severe psychogenic polydipsia generally reduced a tendency to overconsume fluids (as measured by counting the number of fluid restrictions);

2. This was partially due to a combination of aggressive unit restrictions (i.e., level 1, unit restriction due to excessive fluid consumption; and level 2, staff supervised off unit grounds privileges) and internalization of responsible fluid ingestion by each patient due to a combined treatment approach (pharmacological, behavioral management and psycho-educational semiweekly groups);

3. Continuation of the treatment approach required very close perusal, as each SIWI patient's relapse potential without the myriad of resources in place was high. Discharge of the SIWI patients to an "Open Unit" *without rigorous* transitioning procedures would, in the author's opinion, result in the eventual relapse of the patient;

4. A slow, steady increase in fluid access on the locked, SIWI unit, achieved with time and effect of the other treatment interventions, a generalization effect on the mild and moderate SIWI patients, curbing their propensity to overdrink when off the unit. Keeping in mind, this was a "long haul" project, like any other rehabilitation program with a dual diagnosed clientele, a learning curve of "two steps forward and one step back" was expected. It required a thorough examination of each patient's propensity to change a habituated behavior pattern;

5. Careful evaluation of the patients' respective strengths/needs before incorporating any change in the treatment protocol was made at incremental stages. Any facility receiving SIWI patients being discharged from a psychiatric inpatient unit requires a thorough orientation in the current treatment techniques/strategies of this clinical population, in order for a comfortable transition to occur. Consequently, deviation from the treatment protocol could jeopardize the gains made with the SIWI patient;

6. Lastly, an objective assessment instrument evaluating psychogenic polydipsia should be purchased by those facilities attempting to treat psychogenic polydipsia (e.g., Virginia Polydipsia Scale; St. Louis Modified Water Intoxication Scale).

CHAPTER THREE

BEHAVIORAL MANAGEMENT PRINCIPLES AND PROCEDURES: STAFF TRAINING DOCUMENT (MODULES I – VI)

PREAMBLE

Prior to reading the Staff Training Document for treating clients diagnosed with psychogenic polydipsia, a review of the major principles of behavioral modification is presented as a refresher and for those practitioners unfamiliar with this powerful therapeutic approach for treating dysfunctional behavior. The ideal way to use behavioral strategies is within a cooperative venture between the professional and the client. Strategies should be well planned, systematically implemented, and revised to suit changes in the client's behavior or in the demands of the situation. The author gratefully acknowledges the information provided in an excellent training resource in behavioral management, *Behavioral Habilitation Through Proactive Programming* (Bernstein, G.S., Ziarnik, J.P., Rudrud, E.H & Czajkowski, L.A., 1981). The subsequent behavioral management program adapts many of the teaching concepts originally developed in this resource.

BASIC PRINCIPLES OF BEHAVIORAL MANAGEMENT

Operant behavior, in contrast to *respondent behavior*, is under voluntary control. It is influenced and controlled by events or consequences that follow its occurrence. Operant behavior includes all behavior that "operates" on changes or affects the outside environment (Keller, 1969). Almost any movement under the voluntary control of an individual may be appropriately classified as operant behavior. Operant behavior is determined by the conditions or consequences that follow it. Consequences of a response that increase the probability of its occurrence are referred to as reinforcers (Keller, 1969). A *reinforcer* is anything that increases the probability that the response it follows will be emitted again. The response is strengthened by an increase in the frequency of its appearance. When the consequences that follow a response have increased the frequency of that response, *conditioning* has occurred. The strength of a response decreases when reinforcement is terminated. If reinforcement is completely withdrawn for a period of time, the response rate tends to return to the preconditioned rate or operant level. The decrease in response strength is referred to as *extinction* (Reece, 1966).

Operationally defined, a *positive reinforcer* is any stimulus that increases the probability of the response it follows. A *negative reinforcer* may be defined as any stimulus that, by its removal, increases the probability of the response that follows it (Keller, 1969). In positive reinforcement the response is strengthened by the addition of something that follows its occurrence. Positive reinforcers may be grouped into three general categories (1) social reinforcers, (2) tokens and tangible reinforcers, and (3) intrinsic reinforcers. Praise, approval and affection are examples of social reinforcers. Tangible reinforcers refer to material items that can be experienced with the sense, that is, eaten, touched, seen. Food, candy, toys, and games are all examples of tangible reinforcers. Tokens may assume the form of check marks, points, plastic strips, or just about anything that can be exchanged for tangible reinforcers or reinforcing events. Intrinsic reinforcers refer to satisfactions inherent in performing an activity itself. These satisfactions typically involve curiosity, novelty, and pride resulting from achievement. In negative reinforcement response probability is increased because something is removed or withdrawn (Skinner, 1953). The removal or withdrawal of almost any aversive stimulus, after a response to it, typically acts as a negative reinforcer.

Primary reinforcers are stimuli that have biological significance and/or satisfy a physiological need. Thus, water, food, and sexual release may be designated primary reinforcers. *Secondary or conditioned reinforcers* refer to stimuli that have acquired reinforcement properties by being associated or paired with primary reinforcers or stimuli that have established power. Generally, any stimulus that is paired with and precedes a primary reinforcer may acquire secondary reinforcer properties. Consequently, a word or a smile may function as a secondary reinforcer. The stimuli that do, in fact, acquire secondary reinforcement properties are related to a person's life history (Skinner, 1953; Lundin, 1974; Travers, 1977). Stimuli that have been paired with more than one primary reinforcer acquire the attributes of *generalized reinforcers*. These are stimuli that have reinforcement properties regardless of the conditions operative at the time (e.g., money). Money acquires a generalized reinforcement property when it is used to obtain and satisfy primary needs. Other stimuli may also function as generalized reinforcers, since they have frequently been paired with more than one primary reinforcer (e.g., attention, approval, and affection). With the exception of primary reinforcers, stimulus conditions have no inherent capacity to reinforce. The capacity to reinforce is acquired. One cannot assume that certain stimulus conditions will automatically reinforce a person's behavior. *Generalization* is behavior that is learned in one stimulus situation (e.g. A patient diagnosed with psychogenic polydipsia in a locked, inpatient unit) and tends to be expressed in other situations (e.g., patient takes new, appropriate coping strategies learned on the locked unit to a community residence).

As a consequence, one does not have to resort completely to trial-and-error behavior to know how to behave. It is difficult to promote or modify behavior until the behavior to be changed is stated in *operational terms*. An operationally defined change objective (a) is stated in terms that are observable and measurable and (b) specifies the behaviors to be performed and the exact conditions in which they are expected to occur. Differential reinforcement is used to help the learner discriminate and perform appropriate responses. This is done by selectively reinforcing the desired response and omitting reinforcement when an inappropriate response is made. When a person learns to make a particular response in the presence of a specific stimulus, stimulus control has been established.

BASIC PROCEDURES IN CONDITIONING OPERANT BEHAVIOR

At least six basic procedures are considered essential in conditioning operant behavior, they are stated below (Reese, 1966):

1. ***Define and state operationally the behavior to be changed***. The target behavior (i.e., the behavior to be changed) should be described in terms of the observable behavior the client is to perform, the standard(s) by which you will consider the performance acceptable, and the conditions under which the behavior is expected to occur;

2. ***Obtain a baseline or operant level of the behavior that is considered desirable to promote or change***. Once the target behavior has been stated operationally, its frequency or magnitude should be determined before the behavior is reinforced or treated. Subsequently, it should be possible to determine the effects of the treatment and whether any treatment procedures need to be changed;

3. ***Arrange the learning or treatment situation so that the desirable behavior will occur***. Before reinforcement is administered, it is necessary to determine whether the individual can perform the desired response (e.g., client's ability to drink fluids responsibly during the "open water" periods on the hospital unit). To increase the strength or frequency of response (drinking fluids responsibly) it is necessary to determine present performance level (e.g., duration of "open water" access on the unit) and reinforce those responses the client can execute easily. A response in the client's repertoire can often be prompted by a verbal request that specifies the desired behavior and the reinforcement given;

4. ***Identify potential reinforcers***. Before most people will do something, they must want something. With the possible exception of primary reinforcers and some aversive stimuli, a stimulus has no inherent reinforcement property. The reinforcement property of a stimulus must be determined, that is, its capacity to increase response probability. Some stimuli (e.g., attention and affection) function as generalized reinforcers and may often promote the type of response that is desirable. The most useful method for identifying potential reinforcers is to observe a person in free-choice activities;

5. ***Shape and/or reinforce the desired behavior***. If a client is able to perform the desired response (e.g., drink fluids with more responsibility), reinforce it on its first and every subsequent appearance if possible, until it has assumed appropriate strength. Once the response is being performed with *high* frequency, the reinforcement schedule may be changed to ensure its durability (e.g., increasing the duration of the "open water" access on the unit). However, if the client is unable to perform the desired behavior (e.g., drinking fluids responsibly during the "open water" access), successive approximations of the behavior must be identified and appropriately reinforced (e.g., reducing the duration of "open water" access and immediately reinforcing responsible drinking habits at the new reduced duration of time); and

6. ***Maintain records of the reinforced behavior to determine whether response strength or frequency has increased***. To determine whether the reinforcement contingencies have been effective, longitudinal records must be kept. Comparison of each treatment session with the baseline rate (pretreatment) quickly reveal whether the reinforcement has promoted the response considered desirable. If the reinforcement procedures are not producing the desired result, it is necessary to determine why and to make appropriate adjustments.

PREMACK PRINCIPLE

The essence of the Premack Principle is that any low-probability behavior can be reinforced by an opportunity to engage in a high-probability behavior (e.g., the grandmother example—eat your meat and vegetables; then you may have dessert). Homme, Csanyi, Gonzales, and Rechs (1969) developed a systematic set of procedures for enhancing classroom learning that can be applied to clients with mild/moderate psychogenic polydipsia learning to drink fluids more responsibly.

A. Motivation management
1. Specify the desired learning objectives and/or task behaviors (reducing tendency to overdrink any/all fluids); and

2. Identify appropriate reinforcing activities and events (high-probability behaviors).

B. Develop an appropriate instructional program

1. Assess the client's achievement regarding responsible drinking habits with any/all fluids;

2. Prepare individual task assignments (i.e., structured time activities during the day and early evening). During the day, measure the client's drinking habits via weighing procedure QID (4 times daily). Each client should have a progress check to determine sufficient mastery of task objective (responsible drinking habits as measured through weighing four times per day); and,

3. Clearly indicate to the clients the expectations each day by which successful completion of the task is required (i.e., responsible drinking habits).

C. Formulation of a Contract

1. Write in simple terms the task (responsible drinking habits of any/all fluids) to be performed, specifying the amount of work to be done and criteria for successful completion (clients are placed on a token economy reward system which is discussed below);

2. Indicate the reinforcing events for successful completion of each task assignment (clients are placed on a token economy reward system):

   a) Arrange the reinforcing events (RE's) so they are given frequently and immediately upon the execution of the task behavior (e.g., if client complies with the daily treatment objectives they receive a reward);

   b) State the "contract" positively to the client. Use the reinforcing events to promote the desired behavior e.g., Joe, you controlled your drinking today. Here is your reward, and I look forward to you doing the same tomorrow. Avoid the use of negative contingencies to promote the desired behavior.

D. Specify the reinforcing events (RE's) and arrange an RE area in the Unit.

1. Design an RE menu on which highly desirable reinforcing events are listed. The menu should consist of daily program activities for each client;

2. Arrange the RE's in 15-60 minute activities to provide for the variation in each client's structured, daily activities;

3. Encourage the clients to attend the daily programming and to self-monitor their behavior to influence maximum point accumulation on their token economy schedules; and,

4. Use sign-in and sign-out sheets to regulate the RE activities being attended punctually.

E. Implementing the program

1. Show the RE programs to the residents and explain the nature of each program's rationale *vis-à-vis* the resident's increased quality of life;

2. Explain the RE menu (daily schedule of structured programming) and the expectations for completing the program tasks. Discuss progress checks, going to and signing into the RE program with each attendance;

3. Give the clients a "trial run," going through each step of the procedure, such as the client signing the attendance sheet at each programmed activity. When the RE is completed, the instructor makes a progress check. This allows day-to-day observation of each client's successes and failures and provides information re: a "token economy" reward system, daily/weekly/monthly.

STAFF TRAINING DOCUMENT (MODULES I-VI)

PREAMBLE

The following behavioral management curriculum was devised in order to train multidisciplinary team members who work with clients diagnosed with mild, moderate and severe psychogenic polydipsia. The table of contents has been listed prior to the six-module curriculum to allow the reader a quick perusal of the topics germane to behavioral management. The author adapted many of the behavioral approaches found in the previously noted resource (Bernstein, Ziarnik, Rudrud, & Czajkowski, 1981) as they matched the knowledge requirements and methodology essential to work competently with residents diagnosed with this co-occurrent disorder.

TABLE OF CONTENTS

MODULE I
Culture Change in the Work Environment
(Author's comments are indented)

CONCEPTS:
GUIDELINES FOR CHANGE IN AN ORGANIZATION

> **Comment:** Working in a community group home milieu with dual diagnosed clientele requires five core dimensions to be learned by the staff: skill variety, task identity, task significance, feedback, and autonomy.

- **Skill variety:** a comfort in using an array of abilities for the benefit of the client.
- **Task identity:** Understanding/relating a correct set of skills to complete the task at hand.
- **Task significance:** Ability to accurately prioritize a presented task.
- **Feedback:** Providing information promptly.
- **Autonomy:** Ability to work independently.

1. Make a clear commitment to the change effort influenced by a dual diagnosed clinical population.
Change that is mandated is less likely to occur. It is important to work this commitment through with the people actually making the change;

2. Assess readiness and resources.
Planning and conceptual foresight will greatly enhance the change process. Think through key issues and problems;

3. Anticipate potential problems.
Provide for a problem-solving mechanism during the innovation process. A basic expectation of any change process is that it will lead to problems as well as to benefits. Flexibility is the key concept;

4. Involve key staff and potential adopters.
In planning for the innovation it is important to identify and involve key people within the organization who can lead/advocate further change effort. Outside persons cannot and should not assume this role;

5. Provide for outside consultation/training on the adoption process.
Consultation can be helpful in planning the change as well as in dealing with the many problems that will arise during the change process. A consultant can be an important resource for debriefing issues/problems and offering constructive solutions;

6. Create a positive vision for change.

Focus your major efforts on supporting desired behavior rather than on eliminating unwanted behaviors. It is important to be persistent and remain focused on a positive vision of what is needed. Organizational change presents an opportunity for personal change, if we are open to it and if the process of communication is open. If we can express our feelings and concerns and have them responded to, both planned and unplanned changes can be integrated more easily;

> **Comment:** Clients require consistent motivation by the staff. Symptom reduction improves job satisfaction and decreases rate of job turnover by the staff.

7. Consider how you can build individual/organizational enthusiasm and support for the innovation.

The reason you have created for the change effort needs to be communicated to the staff. They need to understand this vision and how it relates to the new direction the organization is taking. Staff members are influenced by emotional appeal as well as its reasonableness, how it will be translated into practice/how this new practice will benefit the clients diagnosed with psychogenic polydipsia;

8. Interpersonal contact between adopters and those leading the change effort.

Contact between the trainer and staff must be substantive, long-term and focused. Lack of adequate support during implementation is a major source of failure in change efforts; and,

9. Evaluate the change effort.

Things to consider: Have the planned changes occurred? Are the effects of these changes as great as or less than what was predicted? Are there any positive or negative unanticipated outcomes? Evaluation information can be fed back into the planning process of the organization and utilized to develop further change.

NORMALIZATION PHILOSOPHY (SIX PRINCIPLES) CONCEPTS (WOLFENSBERGER, 1972)

The principles of normalization refer to ensuring that clients lead a life as close to "normal" as possible. How the behaviors are taught is as important as the behaviors to be taught.

> **Comment:** The staff are change agents performing helping roles.

1. A normal rhythm of the day.

In applying this principle to the client diagnosed with psychogenic polydipsia, make certain that getting up, dressing, attending to hygiene, eating and working times are a reflection of the community norms not a function of staff convenience;

> **Comment:** Clients improve their level of independence by increasing their overall function.

2. A normal rhythm of the week.

Most of us work in one place, sleep in another, and enjoy recreation in another. We see too many programs that utilize one or two places for all activities. Be creative about where you provide programs. Make WHERE related to the norms of your community;

3. A normal development Life cycle.

Correct people who behave as if the clients are children. Make certain programs, methods, and activities reflect age appropriate expectations;

4. A range of choices.

A range of choices should occur at two distinct levels within the program. First, choice for clients needs to occur at a programmatic level. Clients need to be involved as much as possible in choosing goals, methods, or programs (e.g., choosing a reinforcer). Second, clients have needs/ desires. If we never allow clients free choices (dignity of risk)—to go, not go, stay, not stay— how can we expect them make appropriate choices when placed in independent situations;

> **Comment:** "Dignity of risk" provides clients the opportunity to attempt to succeed or fail in an activity.

5. The right to economic standards.

The programs should endeavor to strive to apply technology to clients and to teach marketable skills (e.g., practical as well as recreation centered). Without the skills necessary to access a normal economic existence, the clients will not learn habilitative services nor assimilate a sense of empowerment, and internal locus of control.

WRITING INTEGRATED PLANS OF CARE (IPC)
(BERNSTEIN, ZIARNIK, RUDRUD & CZAJKOWSKI, 1981, SEE CHAPTER 5)

Concepts

Developing *Integrated Plans of Care (IPC'S)* for each client diagnosed with psychogenic poly-dipsia improves training and follows six principles of behavioral management;

1. Coordination of planning and programming IPC's

IPC's are developed by the program staff, as the Integrated Plan of Care is developed the staff can coordinate their efforts to meet the *individualized needs* of the respective client and ensure effective implementation of these plans;

> **Comment:** Grouping by job activity allows staff to work on the same functions and processes regarding the development of personalized plans of care for this unique clinical population. Open-ended thinking and dialogue with clients are encouraged.

2. Development of a sequential plan.

Adapted from Bernstein et al., *Behavioral Habilitation through Proactive Programming.* Copyright © 1981 by Paul H. Brookes Publishing Co., Inc. Baltimore. Used by permission.

"You must know where you are going if you want to get there."

Short-term objectives are intermediate steps between the client's present level of functioning and the accomplishment of longer term goals. As a result, short-term objectives are sequential and relate to increasing levels of complexity and mastery;

3. Specification of individual needs/services.

The IPC planning process focuses attention on the unique needs of a client diagnosed with psychogenic polydipsia. Each team member should consider evaluation results, current level of functioning in educational, vocational and independent living areas, the strengths/needs of the individual and areas of concern expressed by the client, his/her parents and/or guardians. The client's total needs must be addressed in the IPC;

4. Systematic evaluation.

The development of an IPC plan requires both formative (ongoing) and summative (end) evaluation procedures to be in place (i.e., staff training, baseline assessment treatments, posttreatment). Each client should have an annual, formalized evaluation that assesses the effectiveness of the total IPC process;

5. Increased service provider accountability.

The IPC represents a statement of intent among service providers regarding behavioral methods that will assist the client in meeting stated goals/objectives (e.g., reduction of fluid drinking). The written program reduces misunderstanding between the consumers (clients) and the clinical staff because it specifies individual responsibilities for implementing various components of the IPC; and,

> **Comment:** A written program is an accountable measure of evaluation regarding a client's current level of functioning.

6. Improved communication with consumers.

The "consumers" are those individuals who receive services; the client, his or her parents and/or guardians, and the advocates for the client. By having consumers involved in the IPC process, service providers are demonstrating a concern for the outcomes of the IPC process and a concern for the needs of the consumers. The IPC communicates what specific services (via behavioral management principles) are to be provided for each client diagnosed with psychogenic polydipsia, rather than a general statement indicating "a client will be involved in a special program."

COMPONENTS IPC

> **Comment:** The group home continuum attempts to maximize several strategic treatment considerations simultaneously (e.g., behavioral, psychosocial, and medication).

Concepts
An IPC will include the following:

1. Present level of performance regarding each client;

2. Daily, weekly, monthly data collection regarding the client's goal attainment and subsequent receipt or non-receipt of a reward;

3. Measurable and sequential intermediate steps between the client's current level of performance and goal attainment (daily, weekly, monthly goal achievement);

4. Specific services needed to meet the unique needs of each client (e.g., reinforcers for each client are "tailor-made");

5. Projected dates when the program will be initiated (e.g., baseline), daily, weekly, monthly reinforcers to achieve goals to be highlighted per each respective client's progress;

6. Justification of the behavioral management program for the client, then respective movement (i.e., progress) up/down baseline and treatment phases of the program;

7. Specification of the role(s) of the clinical staff for each client's IPC implementation; and,

8. Evaluation procedures, schedules and goal(s), criteria for determining whether each client's daily, weekly, monthly goals were achieved.

Adapted from Bernstein et al., *Behavioral Habilitation through Proactive Programming*. Copyright © 1981 by Paul H. Brookes Publishing Co., Inc. Baltimore. Used by permission.

MODULE II
Operationalizing Terms

Concepts

1. In developing an IPC, it is necessary to develop long-term (three-month) goals and short-term objectives;

2. Operationalized terms are observable and measurable descriptions of the behavior that is expected to be accomplished by each client;

3. Operationalized behavior is not a difficult task. It requires the team to describe what the client must do when the goal(s) is accomplished;

4. Examples of operationalized terms: to complete; to operate; to identify; to count; to name;

5. Important conditions refer to special circumstances surrounding the performance. In general, they reflect the who, what, when, and where of the objectives; and,

6. When writing an operationalized goal it is necessary to specify the difficulty level of the task required by the client (e.g., this refines objectives re: specification).

Comment: Staff must be able to match a treatment task with a client function.

TIME, FREQUENCY, RATE, AND ACCURACY CRITERION

Concepts
Specifying the criteria of mastery allows the clinical staff to know whether the client has accomplished the goals. The most common criteria include time, frequency, rate, and accuracy;

Time
Time is used as a criteria for acceptable performance. Examples include:

1. I will go to weigh scale 4-5 minutes (time period) per day;

2. I will comply with staff re: weigh-ins four times per day.

Frequency
Frequency refers to count (number of times per day, week, month). Often frequency criteria is combined with time criterion (e.g., three times per shift).

Rate

Rate refers to frequency divided by amount of time (e.g., I will complete a task four times within three hours).

Accuracy

Accuracy is expressed in terms of *percentages*. (e.g., I will achieve 90% of tokens per day to have a desired reward).

> **Comment:** Accurately determining which of the four criteria to use in treatment is a basic tenet for successful evaluation.

LONG TERMS GOALS (LTG'S)

Concepts

Long Term Goals (LTG's) have five components:

1. Direction of change;

2. Statement of deficit or excess;

3. A "From" statement;

4. A "To" statement; and

5. Resources needed

> **Comment:** Treatment programs designed for clients with a co-occurrent disorder use sequential interdependence along a continuum to refine the degree of problem solving and to allow close coordination and timing so work flows are smooth. The LTG component system should be learned quickly and effectively by the team. It should reduce treatment error!

1. Direction of Change

Direction of Change refers to what is to be accomplished with the individual's behavior. Three things can be accomplished:

- a) increased;
- b) maintained;
- c) decreased

2. Statement of Deficit or Excess

Deficits refer to behaviors that are to be increased or improved (e.g., following directions, attending to task). *Excessive Behaviors* are behaviors that occur too frequently. Excessive be-

Adapted from Bernstein et al., *Behavioral Habilitation through Proactive Programming*. Copyright © 1981 by Paul H. Brookes Publishing Co., Inc. Baltimore. Used by permission.

haviors are also behaviors that are to be decreased (e.g., incidents of physical aggressiveness; noncompliance; overdrinking any/all fluids).

There are two ways to approach behavioral problems:

- a) Implementation of a program designed to decrease behaviors (e.g., decrease the number of anger outbursts); and
- b) Implementation of a program designed to increase the periods of time between undesirable behaviors (e.g., increase the amount of time between anger outbursts). This second approach requires the use of positive reinforcement techniques and builds on the client's strengths;

3. "From" Statement
The "from" statement is a description of the individual's present level of functioning within the area of deficit or excess (e.g., from being dressed treatment with physical assistance);

4. "To" Statement
The "to" statement refers to the expected level of performance after the program has been implemented. It reflects the goal to be attained (e.g., to comply with instructions within five seconds of being given them); and,

5. Resources Needed
Many objectives require a statement regarding what resources will be needed to accomplish the expected level of performance. The resources by specialists, materials and methods (e.g., use of speech therapy, occupational therapy, recreation therapy, vocational/individual counseling).

Summary of Five Components to Programming LTG's
Statement of Direction + Statement of Deficit/Excess + From Statement + To Statement + Resources Needed = Long-Term Goal

(e.g., Joe will increase his frustration tolerance from being angry periodically throughout the shift to being able to control his anger using appropriate coping strategies).

> **Comment:** Treatment programs should be developed with reciprocal interdependence, which is treatment alignment in each group home.

SHORT TERM GOALS (STG'S)

Concepts

1. Short-term objectives (STG's) are the intermediate steps between the client's present level of functioning and the expected levels of functioning stated in the LTG's;

2. STG's specify intermediate steps between the "from" and "to" statements;

Adapted from Bernstein et al., *Behavioral Habilitation through Proactive Programming.* Copyright © 1981 by Paul H. Brookes Publishing Co., Inc. Baltimore. Used by permission.

3. STG's are operationalized descriptions of the intended outcomes of intervention strategies. They include the criteria by which intervention success is measured;

4. Operational Statements noting important conditions, difficulty level/time, frequency, and accuracy criteria are also included;

5. STG's provide a way of evaluating how the individual is progressing on programs and how well the programs are working;

6. STG's include: operationalized terms methodology levels of performance special resources criteria of acceptable performance.

Comment: Reciprocal interdependence imposes coordination and problem solving requirements that are consistent throughout the group home continuum.

Operationalized Terms

Operationalized Terms are descriptions of behaviors that are:

1. Observable and measurable.

The operationalized behavior should reflect the intended outcome of the intervention strategy;

Comment: Using operational terms helps to standardize information during times of emergency and/or crisis.

2. Methodology

Methodology refers to who will do what, where and when—in other words, how the long-term goal will be accomplished. An appropriate teaching/objective plan is constructed so that any staff member can read the plan and implement the program correctly, even if the staff has had no prior experience with the program;

3. Scheduling

The best philosophy is to program for a small number of new behaviors at a time and, once progress is seen in these behaviors, then add more. Use small steps in your programs (e.g., behaviors to be reinforced increased);

4. Instructions and Cues

When training programs are implemented, staff use instructions and cues to communicate desired behaviors to the clients. KISS—Keep It Simple! When using verbal cues with this clinical population, consider vocabulary used, complexity of instructions, length of verbalization, volume/tone of voice, repetitions, and restatements. * *If a staff member does not communicate instruction with appropriate nonverbal cues, learning is often impeded.*

** *When using nonverbal cues, consider eye contact, smiling, facial gestures, body motions, physical contact, and level of attention before giving the cue to the resident. General cues refer to en-*

Adapted from Bernstein et al., *Behavioral Habilitation through Proactive Programming.* Copyright © 1981 by Paul H. Brookes Publishing Co., Inc. Baltimore. Used by permission.

vironmental cues that set the occasion for a client's behavior to occur. When using general cues, consider physical setting, general rules, physical layout, and social factors.

> **Comment:** This clinical population is most often diagnosed with a co-occurent disorder (e.g., schizophrenia and psychogenic polydipsia), thereby necessitating treatment consistency to augment improved functioning.

Levels of Performance

Specify the criteria for and conditions in which training is to occur. They should address the client's ability in mastering the task and specifically the client's response to prompts. Prompts are levels of assistance provided by the staff member. They may be physical, gestural or verbal in nature.

Physical prompts are those prompts in which the staff physically assists the client in accomplishing a task or behavior.

A *gestural prompt* requires less physical assistance to the client.

A *verbal prompt* provides no physical assistance to the client. The staff member gives verbal cues to the client that will assist the client in completing the task or the behavior.

* Ultimately the client will be able to perform the task independently or with minimal prompts

5. Special Resources

When specifying the procedures that are to be utilized, it is necessary to identify which staff members are to be responsible for accomplishing certain tasks. Additionally, special materials/resources need to be identified; and,

6. Criteria:

Criteria of acceptable performance are used to determine whether the objective has been accomplished. These criteria may include: time, frequency, rate, difficulty level and/or accuracy depending on the objective.

> **Comment:** Proximity control (close, physical presence) often acts as a mediator for clients who have increasing levels of anxiety, then overdrink any/all fluids.

OVERVIEW OF COMPONENTS

Concepts

Using behavioral management principles, the IPC assists the multidisciplinary team in planning and providing services to the clients diagnosed with psychogenic polydipsia. The minimum components should include:

1. Present level of performance;

2. Long-term goals (quarterly);

3. Short-term objectives to achieve each LTG;

4. Specific services needed;

5. Projected dates when any special service will be initiated;

6. Justification for the type of future placements and current services needed;

7. Specifying staff members responsible for implementation of the IPC;

8. Evaluation procedures, schedules, and objective criteria for determining whether LTG's and LTG's were achieved.

Comment: The staff must retain contact across the group home continuum. The greater the rate of staff turnover, the greater the need to provide accurate and consistent information to reduce communication breakdown and turnover potential.

Long-term goals (LTG's) reflect where the client should be <u>within three months</u> of starting the program in the respective Unit they reside.

Each LTG should consist of:

1. Direction of change;

2. A statement of deficit or excess;

3. A "from" statement;

4. A "to" statement;

5. Resources needed.

Short-term objectives (STG's) reflect a sequential progression from the client's present level of performance to the long-term goal.

STG's should consist of:

1. Operationalized terms;

2. Methodology;

Adapted from Bernstein et al., *Behavioral Habilitation through Proactive Programming.* Copyright © 1981 by Paul H. Brookes Publishing Co., Inc. Baltimore. Used by permission.

3. Levels of performance;

4. Special circumstances;

5. Criteria of acceptable performance.

The LTG and STG's are derived from the client's assessment and IPC process.

> **Comment:** Each client's functional strengths and needs impose differing degrees of information processing requirements to facilitate learning success.

It is necessary to know where the individual is prior to setting LTG's

Additionally, STG's must reflect sequential steps between the client's current level of functioning and his/her expected level of functioning. There must be a direct logical relationship between STG's and the LTG's. The LTG should reflect the sum of all of its STG's (see below):

- Operationalized terms + important conditions + criteria of mastery = short-term goal.
- Short term goal 1 + 2 + 3 + 4 = Long Term Goal

Rules to Remember:

1. Effective client programming is the result of the IPC behavior management process;

2. Although the IPC behavioral management process may appear tedious, once the multidisciplinary team member becomes familiar with the process, the amount of time required to develop an IPC decreases and training becomes more efficient. Prior to resident meetings, the multidisciplinary staff should prepare a list of client strengths, needs, and possible goal areas.

MODULE II—HANDOUT #1
(see Bernstein et al., 1981. p. 83)

- When developing the IPC it is necessary to develop long-term goals (LTG's) and short-term objectives (STG's);

- Both goals (ST, LT) need to be stated in operationalized terms;

- Operationalized terms are observable and measurable descriptions of the behavior that is expected to be accomplished;

- Examples of operationalized terms include measurable and observable conditions: to complete, to operate, to define, to name, to identify, to count.

In writing operationalized goals, the criteria for acceptable performance must be considered. Criteria include:

- Difficulty level (what mastery is expected)

- Time (period of time)

- Frequency (count)

- Rate (frequency divided by time)

- Accuracy (percentage)

Important conditions refer to special circumstances surrounding the performance. They include who, what, when, and where.

Adapted from Bernstein et al., *Behavioral Habilitation through Proactive Programming*. Copyright © 1981 by Paul H. Brookes Publishing Co., Inc. Baltimore. Used by permission.

MODULE II—HANDOUT #2

(see Bernstein et al., 1981. p 88)

LONG-TERM GOALS FORMAT (IPC)

Summary

Long-Term Goals have five components in the IPC:

1. Statement of direction of change: *Joe will…*

    +

2. Statement of deficit/excess: *… increase his frustration tolerance…*

    +

3. "From statement": *…from being angry periodically throughout the shift…*

    +

4. "To statement": *…to being able to control his anger throughout the shift…*

    +

5. Resources needed: Using the log with written cues.

= LONG-TERM GOAL

MODULE II—HANDOUT #3
(see Bernstein et al. p. 88)

- Short-term objectives are intermediate steps between the resident's current level of functioning and the expected levels of functioning stated in the long-term goals;

- Short-term objectives specify intermediate steps between the "from" and "to" statements and are operationalized descriptions of the intended outcomes of intervention strategies.

Short-Term Objectives include:

1. Operationalized terms (behaviors that are observable and measurable);

2. Methodology (who, what, where and when);

3. Levels of performance (criteria for conditions in which training occurs);

4. Special resources (certain materials, self, resources required);

5. Criteria of acceptable performance (time, frequency, rate, difficulty level, and/or accuracy).

Adapted from Bernstein et al., *Behavioral Habilitation through Proactive Programming*. Copyright © 1981 by Paul H. Brookes Publishing Co., Inc. Baltimore. Used by permission.

MODULE II – HANDOUT #4

(see Bernstein et al. p. 85 – 87)

LONG-TERM GOAL

Domain: ADL behavior

Joe will increase an appropriate repertoire of ADL skills from:

- a) too long to dress
- b) too verbally abusive
- c) too socially isolated

to:

- a) reduced time to dress
- b) reduced verbal abuse
- c) reduced social isolation

by: STG's

1. 1. Joe will reduce time to dress to five minutes total duration with less than three prompts from the staff per shift over a one-month period;

2. 2. Joe will reduce his verbal abuse to residents/staff to less than five episodes (frequency) per shift by staff's verbal praise for appropriate language each shift for a one-month period;

3. 3. Joe will increase his social interaction with residents by receiving five prompts from staff each shift for a period of one month.

Adapted from Bernstein et al., *Behavioral Habilitation through Proactive Programming*. Copyright © 1981 by Paul H. Brookes Publishing Co., Inc. Baltimore. Used by permission.

MODULE III
(see Bernstein et al. Chapter 6)

Behavior Assessment - Where Are We?

CONCEPTS

What to Measure?
Too often we start programming without performing a careful functional analysis of the behavior.

Functional Analysis
Functional analysis involves identifying the A-B-C of a client's behavioral repertoire.

A = Antecedents are events that occur just before problem behaviors;

B = Behaviors to be modified;

C = Consequences are events that follow problem behaviors.

Anecdotal Records
Clinical staff notes during the shift are written descriptions of the client's behavior of interest to modify, which includes the antecedents and consequences. The notation should include: who is present; and time, place and nature of task or activity. Be specific and do not use judgemental statements.

Operational Definitions of Behavior
* Define the client's behavior in specific or operational terms. An *operational definition* is one that uses observable and measurable terms;
* In order for a definition to be observable, it must describe not only the behavior to be observed, but also the conditions under which it occurs;
* Specifically, your definition should include: who is doing what, when, how, (and where): e.g.,

* Who: Joan
* What: going on break independently
* When: 10:15 – noon
* How: stop work at break time, travel to Penn Hall at...
Return at …

    Comment: Specific information augments information processing by the client.

DIMENSIONS OF BEHAVIOR

There are FIVE dimensions of behavior:

- Frequency
- Duration
- Latency
- Form
- Intensity

Comment: Specific information facilitates each client's treatment protocol from a strategic, behavioral approach.

1. Frequency
Frequency is defined as how many times a behavior occurs while you are observing it. Before you compare frequencies obtained across several different observation periods, you need to convert the frequency to rates. Rate is defined as frequency divided by length of observation. The rationale for converting frequencies to rates is to observe periods that are not all the same length—the frequencies obtained are not directly comparable;

2. Duration
Duration is how long a behavior lasts;

3. Latency
Latency is how long it is between the presentation of a stimulus and the beginning of the response to it. It is most often measured with respect to compliance;

4. Form
Form is a measure of accuracy; we want to know if the observed behavior meets certain standards for form (e.g., accuracy of bed making); and,

5. Intensity
Intensity is a 3-5 point rating scale, which is most often used to measure effect (e.g., speech volume). Quality of a behavior is a combination of two or more dimensions of behavior. One common combination is that of rate and form (e.g., a sufficient number of…in a given period of time will have an accuracy of…).

Recording Behavior
Once the dimension of behavior has been chosen to measure, you need to decide how to measure it!

Continuous Event Recording
Continuous Event Recording is recording every occurrence of the behavior during a specified

period. You could be recording frequency, duration, intensity, latency, form or some combination of these variables. Event recording is most often used to measure behavior with a clear beginning and ending (e.g., getting dressed);

Interval Recording
Interval recording involves dividing a period of time into short, equal intervals. These intervals are typically from 10 seconds to two minutes long. Then, once per interval, you record whether or not the behavior you are observing occurred. This procedure is often used to measure behaviors that do not have clear beginnings/endings or that vary in duration (e.g., overdrinking any/all fluids). On-task behaviors often do not have clear beginnings and endings;

Time Sampling
Time sampling is utilized when behaviors occur so frequently that it is not practical to observe them during the entire period of interest. More specifically, time sampling involves measuring behavior during each of several short-time periods within the larger period of interest. There are two types:

Random Time Sampling
Random time sampling divides the period during which the behavior of interest occurs into separate short time intervals, usually 5-15 minutes long. Then you decide how many samples per period you want to take and choose that many at random from the total list;

Systematic Time Sampling
Systematic time sampling decides how many time samples you need for each period of interest and how long each sample will be. Then systematically choosing the time each sample will be taken by arranging for the samples at the various times of the day in which you are interested and in all settings of interest. Time samples can be used with either continuous event recording or interval recording.

There are four possible ways of recording behavior:
a) Continuous event recording during the entire period of interest;
b) Interval recording during the entire period of interest;
c) Continuous event recording during time samples, and;
d) Interval recording during time samples.

Examples:

Continuous Event Recording
Recording the length of every temper outburst a client displays at any time;

Interval Recording
Every two minutes during every break and lunch period at the workshop record whether or not a client is socializing;

Continuous Event Recording

During each of four 30-minute samples every day, two of which are taken at "vocational" on weekdays, record whether a client's speech is too loud, too soft, or acceptable each time they speak;

Interval Recording During Time Samples

For the first five minutes of every hour during the working day, record at the end of every 30 seconds whether or not a client is "on task."

ISSUES IN MEASURING/RECORDING BEHAVIOR

Concepts

Observer Drift

Over time observers recording data tend to change the way they apply the definition of the behavior they observe. Hence, agreement should be checked throughout a measurement period to determine whether observer drift is occurring.

Expectancy

Observers may record behavior as changing in the direction they expect, even though the change expected is not happening. This is not "faking" data, people affected by expectancy record what they honestly believe they have seen. Inter-observer agreement (i.e., another person observing) will reduce the tendency of expectancy drift.

Observer Agreement

Inter-observer agreement is calculated as follows:

Frequency Measures – the formula is:

> Smaller frequency X 100 = % agreement of larger frequency
> (For example, Joe recorded the client attending to task 20 times in one hour, and Jill recorded 14 times in another one-hour period of time during the day.
> 14/20 X 100 = 70% agreement;

Duration – the formula is:

> Shorter duration X 100 = % agreement longer duration.

Interval Recording – the formula is:

> Total # agreements X 100 = % agreements divided by (/) Total # agreements + total # disagreements

Observer Agreements can be measured using the same formula as the interval recording formula. The respectable standard for agreement is considered around 90%. Observer agreement should be checked when you begin measuring a behavior and then checked regularly throughout the measurement period.

REPORTING BEHAVIOR – DRAWING GRAPHS TO RECORD BEHAVIOR

(see Bernstein et al. pp. 116-121)

Concepts

A graph is simply a picture of data. A well-made graph provides a descriptive picture that summarizes the measurements you have obtained, a picture that is clear, simple and explicit. Always use a pencil (it's a lot easier and neater to fix a mistake). The specific steps in making a graph are:

1. Draw the Axes

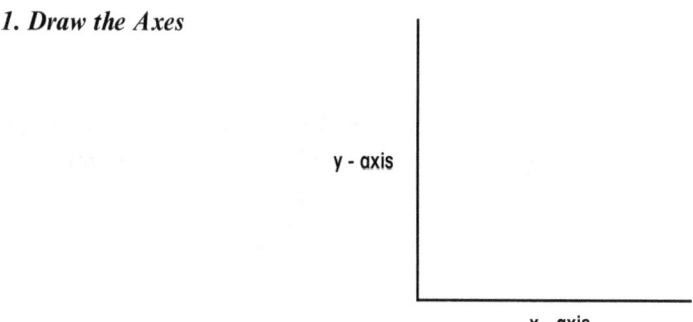

2. Label the Axes. When you graph behavioral data, the X axis is usually time and the Y axis is usually the particular dimensions of behavior you are measuring. Labels should be specific, not general.

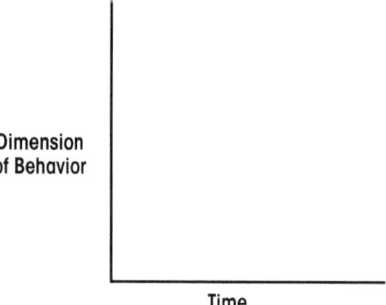

3. Mark the Scales. Since the scales should be equal intervals, the easiest way to develop an accurate graph is to use graph paper.

4. Label the Scales. Use similar divisions on the two axes so that changes in behavior will not appear distorted.

5. Plot Your Data. For each day (or each unit of time period used), go to that day on the horizontal axis and then go up until you are directly to the right of the observed data (or duration) on the vertical axis.

6. Separate and Label Treatment Conditions (A-B design)

A = baseline data (no treatment)

B = treatment data (treatment implemented)

*Correlation does not equal a cause-effect relationship

   Baseline Phase Collect data but no treatment.

   Treatment Phase Treatment implemented and data collection continued as in the baseline phase.

7. Connect the Data Points Within Each Condition. (baseline phase, treatment phase).

8. Title the Graph. The title should be a concise description of what you have graphed.

9. Interpreting the Graphs. Once you have graphed your data, you will need to interpret them. Did the behavior you observed meet the criteria for success? Has the program resulted in any change in behavior? Changes can occur in level, direction, and variability.

(a) Change in **Level**

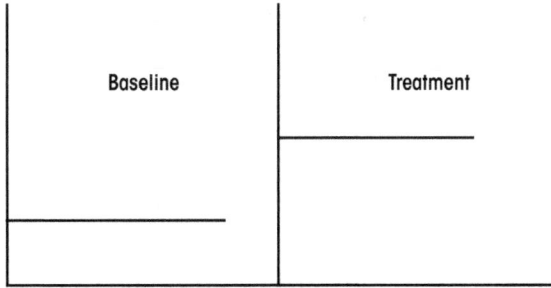

(b) Change in **Direction**

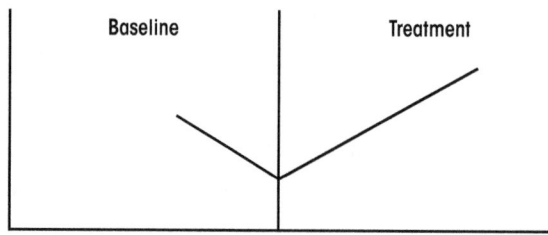

(c) Change in **Variability**

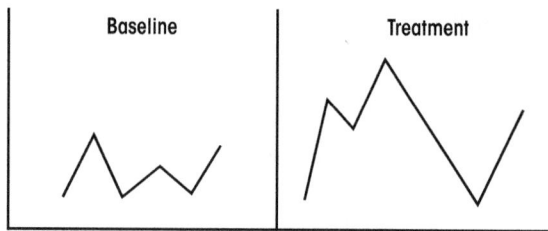

(d) Delayed change in **Level**

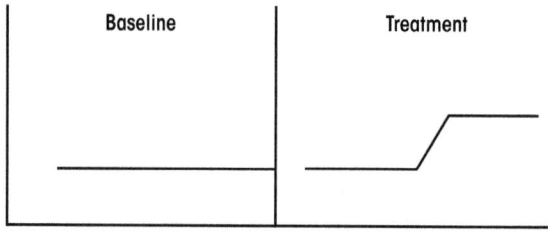

(e) Temporary change in **Direction**

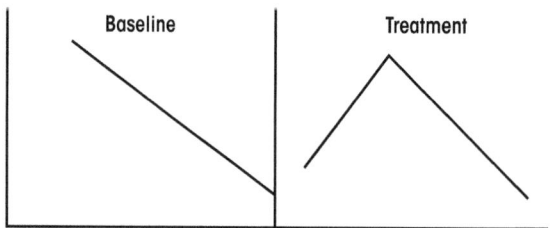

Comment: Graphing the data of each client's functional capabilities should become second nature and be used as an adjunct to support clinical decisions!

Adapted from Bernstein et al., *Behavioral Habilitation through Proactive Programming.* Copyright © 1981 by Paul H. Brookes Publishing Co., Inc. Baltimore. Used by permission.

CHOOSING MEASUREMENTS, RECORDING AND REPORTING PROCEDURES

Concepts

The guidelines below are designed to provide you with a system for selecting appropriate assessment procedures. The Measurement Procedure Form (see Module III- Handout #1) is designed to give you a quick and comprehensive description of your procedures once you have selected them.

Guidelines for Selecting Assessment Procedure

1. Take anecdotal records of client's behavior(s);

2. Operationally define the behavior(s) being assessed;

3. Identify the relevant dimension of the behavior(s);

    a) If how often the behavior occurs is relevant, the dimension is frequency;

    b) If how long the behavior occurs is relevant, the dimension is duration;

    c) *If how long after the cue* is presented the behavior occurs is relevant, the dimension is latency;

    d) *If how well the behavior conforms to a set standard* is relevant, the dimension is form; and,

    e) If how much of the behavior occurs is relevant, the dimension is intensity.

Comment: If the aim of treatment is to help the client achieve a maximum level of independence, then the success of treatment is judged in terms of the goals set for that client.

Select the Recording Procedure

Decide when to observe:

1. Choose continuous recording if the behavior has a clear beginning and ending; choose interval recording if the behavior does not have a clear beginning and ending and if precise duration is not a major concern;

2. If using interval recording, choose the length of the interval, shorter intervals for shorter behaviors, longer intervals for longer, more continuous behaviors. In most cases, choose intervals no less than 10 seconds and no more than 120 seconds in length (except time sampling);

3. Identify all times that the behavior may occur, on all days of the week. Then decide

Adapted from Bernstein et al., *Behavioral Habilitation through Proactive Programming*. Copyright © 1981 by Paul H. Brookes Publishing Co., Inc. Baltimore. Used by permission.

which time sampling is necessary because of high frequency or long duration over long periods, or lack of observer time;

4.   When using time sampling, choose the number of time samples—per day and per week. Come as close as practical to having one sample for each period when the behavior may occur;

5.   Choose the length of the time samples. Consider availability of observer (i.e., nurses, health care workers), difficulty of recording procedures, frequency of behavior;

6.   Choose times for time samples that are representative of the periods of most clinical interest. You may want to observe the behavior continuously for a day or two to identify those periods;

7.   Decide the length of the baseline. Pick a set length in advance and never have less than three observation periods;

a) Determine who will do the observing. Choose the multidisciplinary team members available in the settings selected;

b) Determine where observations are to occur by identifying all settings where the behavior occurs and choosing from those setting and the ones in which it is practical to observe;

c) Identify and locate the tools needed to record observations:

1. Data sheet;

2. Frequency: hand or wrist watch;

3. Duration or latency: stop watch;

4. Interval recording: audible timer;

d) Describe how to record;

1. Design a graph for the data;

2. Design a procedure for assessing inter-observer agreement;

3. Check your procedures to see if anything more can be done to minimize the reactivity of observations. Ask yourself:

a) Are you assessing observer agreement throughout the measurement period to check for observer drift?

b) Is at least one of the observers not involved in implementing the behavior change program to control for expectancy?

c) Is it possible to avoid telling observers when their agreement is being checked?

d) Are the observations as unobtrusive as possible?

8. Arrange to train the observers to use the chosen procedure training for self-monitoring;

9. Review all procedures and make sure that they are as simple as possible.

Comment: Multidisciplinary input on assessment selection becomes a standard operating procedure. Staff evaluation of client behavior should become more accurate and precise with continuous practice and feedback from the team.

Adapted from Bernstein et al., *Behavioral Habilitation through Proactive Programming*. Copyright © 1981 by Paul H. Brookes Publishing Co., Inc. Baltimore. Used by permission.

MODULE III—HANDOUT #1
MEASUREMENT PROCEDURE FORM

(see Bernstein et al. p.135)

Person to be observed _____

Operational definition of behavior to be observed_____

Dimension of behavior to be observed _____

When to observe

    a) days of week _____
    b) times of day_____
    c) dates _____

Who observes_____

Where to observe_____

Tools needed:

    a) data sheet – attach to form
    b) other – include location of each item_____

How to record _____

Graph – attach to form

Procedures for assessing inter observer agreement_____

_____

Procedures for minimizing reactivity_____

_____

Procedures for training observers _____

_____

MODULE III—HANDOUT #1A
ANECDOTAL RECORD FORM

(see Bernstein et al. p. 128)

Resident _____

Observer: _____

Date: _____

TIME

ANTECEDENTS	BEHAVIOR	CONSEQUENCES	LOCATION

TIME

ANTECEDENTS	BEHAVIOR	CONSEQUENCES	LOCATION

TIME

ANTECEDENTS	BEHAVIOR	CONSEQUENCES	LOCATION

MODULE III—HANDOUT # 2
BEHAVIOR OBSERVER FORM

Rate

(see Bernstein et al. p. 129)

DATE

BEHAVIOR	LOCATION	RESIDENT	OBSERVER

Rate

Time Observation Began _____

Time Observation Ended _____

Number of Occurrences _____

MODULE III—HANDOUT # 3
BEHAVIOR OBSERVATION FORM

Duration

(see Bernstein et al. p.130)

DATE

BEHAVIOR	LOCATION	RESIDENT	OBSERVER

Duration

Time Observation Began _____

Time Observation Ended _____

Time Behavior Started _____

Time Behavior Stopped _____

MODULE III—HANDOUT # 4
BEHAVIOR OBSERVATION FORM

Latency

(see Bernstein et al. p. 131)

DATE

BEHAVIOR	LOCATION	RESIDENT	OBSERVER

Latency

Time Observation Began _____

Time Observation Ended _____

Time Cue Given_____

Time Behavior Started Latency _____

MODULE III— HANDOUT # 4A
BEHAVIOR OBSERVATION FORM

Latency

(see Bernstein et al. p. 131)

DATE

BEHAVIOR	LOCATION	RESIDENT	OBSERVER

Time Observation Total # Began _____

Time Observation Total # Ended _____

Total # Began Ended _____

Completed that are correct _____

MODULE III—HANDOUT # 5
BEHAVIOR OBSERVATION FORM

Intensity

(see Bernstein et al. p. 133)

DATE

BEHAVIOR	LOCATION	RESIDENT	OBSERVER

Code:

TL = too loud

TS = too soft

OK = acceptable

NT = not talking

Time   Code   Time   Code

_____

_____

_____

_____

_____

MODULE III—HANDOUT # 6
BEHAVIOR OBSERVATION FORM

Interval Recording

(see Bernstein et al. p. 132)

Date _____

Behavior _____

Resident _____

Observer _____

Behavior Observed _____ Location _____

Length of Intervals _____ seconds

Time Started _____

Adapted from Bernstein et al., *Behavioral Habilitation through Proactive Programming.* Copyright © 1981 by Paul H. Brookes Publishing Co., Inc. Baltimore. Used by permission.

MODULE IV
Behavior Management – How Do We Get There?

(see Bernstein et al. Chapters 7-8)

Concepts

The previous description of how to set up a comprehensive behavioral management program for clients diagnosed with psychogenic polydipsia has provided detailed instruction to achieve positive rather than negative results. The focus has been on the outcome of service, particularly the observation and analysis of observable client changes, in relation to the staff's actions and other external influences (e.g., family; community agencies). The client's functional skills have been evaluated and individualized programs developed that are observable, measurable and training friendly. The following overview demonstrates the areas covered thus far.

BEHAVIOR PRINCIPLES

Module I introduced the first approach to behavioral management programming: it is proactive. That is, a planned rather than a crisis-oriented approach.

Modules II and III introduced the second and third major aspects of the approach: (a) it is individualized to each respective client. The IPC's behavioral management program is fit to the client, not the client to programs; (b) behavioral management is data based—we measure what we do and change it if it isn't working.

Behavioral Management – How Do We Get There?
Module IV introduces you to the fourth aspect of developing IPC's: it is behavioral. We can have an effect on what comes before a task (antecedents), what comes after a task (consequences) and task structure.

A.B.C. MODEL OF BEHAVIOR

The A.B.C. Model of Behavior provides us with a framework for deciding how behaviors can be *modified*. It assumes that behavior is influenced by events on the hospital units/living accommodations for the clients. Events that occur immediately before a behavior are called *antecedents* and events that immediately follow a behavior are called *consequences*.

The entire multidisciplinary team examines the relationships between a behavior and its antecedents and consequences in order to identify those stimuli that may control behavior. More specifically, antecedents may set the occasion for the occurrence of behavior (stressors in the group home precipitate overdrinking and SIWI), and consequences serve to either increase, maintain or decrease a behavior (water intoxication reduces feelings of stress).

Positive consequences that follow a behavior can include events such as attention, praise, tokens, food, or the removal of a negative event such as revoked weekend privileges being lifted.

Negative consequences can be typically unfavorable events, such as reprimands, or the removal of something positive, such as attention and response cost in the token economy.

Antecedents or cues are those events in the environment that set the occasion for a behavior. By observing that certain behaviors are regularly preceded by certain cues, you can systematically alter cues in order to change behavior. For example, the presence of a staff person cueing "on-task" behavior may reduce the tendency for a resident to seek out and overdrink any/all fluids.

The use of *positive reinforcement* is also consistent with the proactive philosophy because it forces programming to focus on what we want the client to do. A *reinforcer* is defined as anything that is presented after a behavior that increases the probability that the behavior will occur again. This means that reinforcement is highly individualized and based on the client's likes and dislikes. Literally, it is anything that works. You cannot decide automatically what will be reinforcing for another person. You must assess a client's likes and dislikes.

CLASSES OF POSITIVE REINFORCEMENT

(a) Primary Reinforcement

Primary reinforcements are rewards pertaining to biological functioning. These include; warmth, sex, comfort and safety.

(b) Secondary Reinforcer

There are two things to remember about secondary reinforcers:

(a) they are generalized from primary reinforcers; and

(b) their reinforcing properties are acquired via learning. For example, the client comes into the world needing/liking food; we have to learn to value the importance of secondary reinforcers such as money, recreation or social interaction.

SECONDARY REINFORCERS

(a) Ask the client what he/she likes;

(b) Observe what the client does—Premack principle. Behavior can be divided into high probability and low probability behaviors. High probability behaviors are those things that an individual, if left to their own devices, will often do. Low probability behavior is something that a person does not do very often. Premack principle theorizes that high probability behavior could be utilized as reinforcers for low probability behaviors (e.g., smoking influencing social interaction).

Reinforcer sampling occurs when individuals are given the opportunity to engage in a number of activities. They are then allowed to make choices about which reinforcers are preferred.

(c) Definition – Try something with a client and see if it works. If you continually present an object, an event, or an activity after a desired behavior and the frequency of that behavior increases, then your consequence is reinforcing. In all cases, remember that reinforcement is defined by its effect on behavior. If the behavior does not change in the way you want it to change, there is a high probability that your consequence is not a reinforcer for that particular individual.

SCHEDULE OF REINFORCERS

Some factors that are important when working with this clinical population include the schedule of reinforcement, the amount of reinforcement, and timing of reinforcement. When the reinforcer delivered is as important as what is delivered. The schedule of reinforcement refers to the relationship between the behavior emitted and the frequency of reinforcement. Careful thought must be given to the schedule of reinforcement whenever a program designed to increase behavior is implemented.

1) Continuous Reinforcement Schedule (CRF)
Every time a desired response is produced, reinforcement is given. The relationship of behavior to reinforcement is 1:1. Skill acquisition is rapid when a behavior is continuously reinforced and should be implemented when teaching a new behavior;

2. Fixed Reinforcement Schedule (F.R.R; F.I.R)
A fixed schedule is closely related to a continuous schedule; for every set of responses or period of time, reinforcement occurs. Whereas a continuous schedule has a behavior-to-reinforcement ratio of 1:1, that of a fixed schedule might be 5:1; 2:1; or 20:1. In any event it is fixed. Two variations on a fixed schedule are:

(a) *Fixed Ratio (F.R)* – for every 2nd, 4th, 7th, etc., behavior, a reinforcer will be delivered;

(b) *Fixed Interval (F.I)* – whereas ratio refers to behavior, interval refers to time. e.g., client "weigh-ins" are on a fixed interval schedule (e.g., 4 times per day: 7:30 a.m., 11:30 a.m., 3 p.m., 7:30 p.m.) at which time a daily reward may be obtained for appropriate weight.

3. Variable Reinforcement Schedule
Two different types of variable schedules are:

(a) Variable interval (V.I) – the amount of time between reinforcement is varied;

(b) Variable ratio (V.R) – the number of times the behavior must be emitted prior to reinforcement is varied.

Variable reinforcement schedules differ from fixed schedules in that there is a changing pattern to the schedule. Some but not all responses are reinforced. A variable schedule might be two responses before reinforcement, then six responses before reinforcement, then one response, then no response etc. In short, the client cannot depend on exactly when reinforcement is coming. Variable reinforcement has the advantage of serving to maintain a behavior for long periods of time without reinforcement.

In regards to overdrinking any/all fluids, behaviors on a variable schedule are more resistant to the loss of reinforcement. A client seeking and finding enough fluids to overdrink on a regular basis becomes very conditioned to self-induced water intoxication and very resistant to changing the behavior, which is very reinforcing. Conversely, to increase a skill or an array of skills that are beneficial to the client, change from continuous to variable reinforcement by gradually reducing the density or frequency of reinforcement. The major rule in reducing the reinforcer density is to believe in the behavior. That is, if performance begins to decrease, the density of reinforcement is being reduced too quickly.

GUIDELINES FOR USING REINFORCERS

1. Reinforce Consistently
Regardless of how reinforcement is delivered, continuously or intermittently, it is necessary to reinforce consistently and specify the behavior to be reinforced;

2. Reinforce Improvements
When a client is asked to do something new or difficult they should be reinforced for progress. DO NOT wait for final accomplishment of the target behavior; reinforce small steps;

3. Pair Verbal Praise with Tangible Reinforcement
Whenever tangible reinforcers are provided, pair verbal praise with the delivery of the reinforcer. Occasionally, verbal praise is not effective; this is especially true with lower-functioning clients diagnosed with psychogenic polydipsia.

However, by pairing verbal praise with the delivery of tangible reinforcers, verbal praise can acquire reinforcing properties. Verbal praise becomes a secondary or acquired reinforcer. Once verbal praise has acquired reinforcing properties, new behaviors can be taught and maintained by its user;

4. Reinforce Immediately
Reinforcement is most effective when delivered immediately after the performance. The short-

Adapted from Bernstein et al., *Behavioral Habilitation through Proactive Programming*. Copyright © 1981 by Paul H. Brookes Publishing Co., Inc. Baltimore. Used by permission.

er the delay between the behavior and the reinforcement, the more effect the reinforcement will have on the behavior.

Delay of reinforcement may result in the accidental reinforcement of an undesired behavior. For example, during the morning, a client engages in a lot of undesirable behaviors. At lunchtime, a staff member sees the client and praises him for being very helpful. The behaviors that were reinforced were the undesirable behaviors rather than helpful behaviors. Delivering reinforcement immediately prevents accidental reinforcement of undesirable behaviors.

Decreasing Behaviors

Intervention procedures that are designed to decrease or eliminate excessive behaviors include:

1. Reinforcing alternative behaviors;

2. Differential reinforcement of other behaviors;

3. Extinction;

4. Timeouts;

5. Response cost; and,

6. Overcorrection

These procedures apply to both appropriate and inappropriate behaviors.

REINFORCING ALTERNATIVE BEHAVIORS

A procedure in which reinforcement is provided for an explicit behavior or behaviors that are incompatible with the target behavior to be decreased.

A list of alternative behaviors that could be reinforced is shown below:

Inappropriate Behaviors

1. Off task

2. Wandering around

3. Aggression, hitting, pushing

4. Noncompliance

Alternate Behaviors

1. Working on task in the room

2. Staying at the work station/sitting at the table

3. Interacting appropriately with others, working on task

4. Compliance with requests, cooperating with others, working on task

Advantages

It is a positive and constructive approach. Since it is a positive reinforcing procedure, it increases appropriate behaviors. For every excessive behavior, there is a related deficit. With this procedure the client receives reinforcement for increasing appropriate behavior.

Disadvantages

It takes time for the appropriate behavior to replace the inappropriate behavior. Until the appropriate behavior is produced at a fairly high rate, the client diagnosed with psychogenic polydipsia still has time available to engage in the inappropriate behavior.

DIFFERENTIAL REINFORCEMENT OF OTHER BEHAVIOR (DRO)

Reinforcement is delivered to the client as long as he or she does not engage in the behavior to be eliminated (e.g., overdrinking fluids). Reinforcement is contingent on the nonoccurrence of a behavior. DRO is different than reinforcing alternative behaviors. In DRO, reinforcement is delivered on a schedule for the nonoccurrence of a target behavior (e.g., overdrinking any/all fluids). Reinforcing alternative behaviors provides reinforcement for the occurrence of the behavior that is incompatible with the target behavior.

Advantages of DRO

DRO is a positive approach because the client receives positive reinforcement when not engaging in the target behavior (i.e., overdrinking any/all fluids). Since the client is not physically removed from the training session, the client has further opportunity to earn reinforcement for engaging in appropriate behaviors. DRO procedures produce rapid decrements in behavior, and the results are very long lasting.

Disadvantages of DRO

DRO requires that reinforcement must be carefully scheduled at first. The time interval for delivering reinforcement should be kept short, allowing the client to earn frequent reinforcement. As inappropriate behavior (e.g., overdrinking any/all fluids) decreases in frequency, which takes a long time (duration), the reinforcement intervals are gradually lengthened. This can be a challenging exercise with this clinical population! Another disadvantage is that the "other" behavior may be worse. The DRO procedure provides reinforcement to the client for engaging in an infinite variety of behaviors other than the specified target behavior. As a result, the client may be engaged in an inappropriate behavior that is not the target behavior when reinforcement is delivered. To reduce this problem, place several of the client's more serious behaviors on DRO simultaneously or by utilizing another reductive procedure.

EXTINCTION

Extinction refers to a procedure in which reinforcement is no longer presented after a behavior has occurred; as a result the behavior decreases. Extinction procedures become extremely effective when combined with positive reinforcement procedures.

Advantages of Extinction
The effects are long lasting, it is an uncomplicated procedure, it is easy to implement, and it does not involve the use of adverse consequences.

Disadvantages of Extinction
Extinction procedures are not designed to strengthen adaptive behaviors. More specifically, when a client exhibits an inappropriate behavior, the staff might ignore the behavior. By doing nothing more than ignoring, the staff does not allow the client to engage in appropriate behavior. Reinforcing events may be difficult to control. One needs to have control over the reinforcers in order to engage in appropriate behavior.

When an extinction procedure is implemented, a client may overdrink any/all fluids. These symptoms may show a temporary increase (response burst) in frequency and/or intensity. An extinction procedure alone usually produces a gradual decrease in the behavior rather than a quick decline. If a quick decrease is desired as with certain aggressive or self-injurious behaviors, it is necessary to combine an extinction procedure with other behavior change procedures or use a different procedure altogether.

SPONTANEOUS RECOVERY

Spontaneous recovery is the re-appearance of a behavior that has been extinguished. It is necessary for the clinical staff to continue to ignore the behavior, if they do not the behavior will be intermittently reinforced (attention is a reinforcing agent). Thus, the behavior will be more likely to occur again because intermittently reinforced behavior is more resistant to extinction. Of Note: Ignoring self-induced water intoxication creates a problem. If the client becomes SIWI it requires immediate seclusion and staff regulation of any/all fluid intake.

TIME-OUT (FROM POSITIVE REINFORCEMENT)

Time-out is a procedure in which the opportunity to earn reinforcers is removed for a *brief* period of time following the occurrences of an inappropriate behavior.

Adapted from Bernstein et al., *Behavioral Habilitation through Proactive Programming*. Copyright © 1981 by Paul H. Brookes Publishing Co., Inc. Baltimore. Used by permission.

Two Types of Time-out Procedures

1. Time-out from positive reinforcement without isolation; and,

2. Time-out from positive reinforcement with isolation.

Time-out without isolation is utilized when the behavior is not harmful, dangerous, or disruptive to other people or is not self-destructive. The difference between time-out without isolation and extinction is that in extinction one specific behavior that has previously been reinforced is no longer reinforced. In time-out, no response is reinforced for a specified period of time following the occurrence of an inappropriate behavior.

Time-out with isolation refers to a procedure in which the client with psychogenic polydipsia is removed from the reinforcing environment (e.g., open unit with access to water). If a client exhibits an inappropriate behavior(s) (e.g., compulsively seeking any/all fluids to over-drink or hostility to other clients and staff) the client is removed to an area where he or she will not disrupt others and where there is nothing to do.

GUIDELINES FOR TIME-OUT PROCEDURES

1. Before utilizing time-out with isolation, try other procedures designed to decrease behavior(s). Time-out is not a positive approach in that the client diagnosed with psychogenic polydipsia has no opportunity to be reinforced for appropriate behaviors while in time-out;

2. Closely monitor how often a client is placed in time-out (i.e., time, date, duration, reason etc.,) and how often the time-out area is utilized. Excessive use of time-out indicates that the training environment is not positively reinforcing;

3. Communicate to other members of the multidisciplinary team and client what behavior will result in the implementation of the time-out contingencies. Consistency in program implementation is essential for decreasing behaviors. Describing the behaviors that result in time-out to the client specifies the relationship between these behaviors and the contingent consequences;

4. Administer time-out in a matter-of-fact, non-emotional manner. Scolding and reprimanding the client are to be avoided, as are requesting apologies, explaining why the client has to go into time-out and praising the resident for going into time-out;

5. Ensure the time-out is time away from positive reinforcement; and,

6. Keep the time-out period short. Time-out periods are generally most effective with periods of less than 30 minutes.

Adapted from Bernstein et al., *Behavioral Habilitation through Proactive Programming*. Copyright © 1981 by Paul H. Brookes Publishing Co., Inc. Baltimore. Used by permission.

Advantages of time-out

A major advantage of time-out is that it is effective in reducing a wide variety of inappropriate behaviors (e.g., temper outbursts, off-task behaviors, hitting, verbal abuse, noncompliance) that are exhibited by clients diagnosed. Time-out produces fairly rapid decrements in behavior and it is a long-lasting procedure.

Disadvantages of time-out

Time-out can be a time-consuming process. It can be abused for a least two reasons. The clinical staff can occasionally forget that time-out must be time-out from reinforcement and that the environment must not be reinforcing for time-out to be effective.

RESPONSE COST

Response cost refers to a procedure in which privileges, tokens, or other reinforcers are removed contingent upon the occurrence of specific inappropriate behaviors (e.g., overdrinking any/all fluids). In other words, inappropriate behaviors *cost* the client privileges, tokens or other reinforcers.

Advantages of Response Cost

The response-cost procedure produces rapid decreases in behaviors that are long lasting. It is usually easier and less disruptive to implement than time-out. It allows the resident to stay in the training environment, where appropriate behavior can be reinforced.

Disadvantages of Response Cost

Determining the size of the response-cost fine. The client must have a reinforcer reserve. The fine should be large enough to decrease the behavior. If the "response cost" removes half of the tokens, the fine is too large. Alternatively, if the client is fined many times during the day, the size of the "response cost" finance is probably too small. It is necessary to provide an opportunity for the client to obtain the lost reinforcers.

To implement a "response cost" procedure, the staff members should record the fine and collect the fine (response cost) as soon as the client has reinforcers available. If the client is continually "in the hole" the response-cost procedure will become ineffective in that reinforcement will never be obtained for appropriate behaviors. This can result in an "it doesn't matter" attitude.

OVERCORRECTION

Overcorrection is a procedure designed to decrease behaviors. It has two basic components: a) to overcorrect the environmental effects of an inappropriate act; and b) to require the disrupter to intensively practice overly correct forms of relevant behavior.

a) Restitutional Overcorrection

Adapted from Bernstein et al., *Behavioral Habilitation through Proactive Programming*. Copyright © 1981 by Paul H. Brookes Publishing Co., Inc. Baltimore. Used by permission.

The client restores the environment to a better state than before the inappropriate behavior occurred. For example, a client who throws work materials would be required to pick up and sort out all the materials and to dust and clean the area; and,

b) *Positive Practice* Positive practice entails repeated practice of a positive behavior. For example, if a client slams a door, regardless of its location, he/she is required to appropriately open and close the door a pre-determined number of times (e.g., three).

Advantages of Overcorrection

Overcorrection has been demonstrated to produce rapid and long- lasting effects. Generally, overcorrection produces more rapid and long-lasting effects than other procedures. It teaches the individual an appropriate behavior through repeated practice.

Disadvantages of Overcorrection It is a time consuming procedure. It must be instituted immediately following the occurrence of an inappropriate behavior. It requires an almost 1:1 staffing/client ratio. Additionally, a client in the overcorrection procedure for a set period of time disallows staff to do other work activities. This technique might be difficult to implement if the client is SIWI!

GUIDELINES FOR USING BEHAVIORAL DECREMENT PROCEDURES

1. Evaluate Environmental Conditions

Often inappropriate or maladaptive behaviors occur as a result of environmental conditions (e.g., when the client was engaged in appropriate staff behaviors, staff did not reinforce him/her);

2. Be Specific

It is necessary to operationalize the behavior that is to be reduced. This is completed so that all staff knows when client X does Y then consequences Z must follow. This also means that consequence Z only occurs when client X completes Y;

3. Be Immediate

The most effective learning occurs when positive or negative consequences immediately follow a behavior. It is important to establish the functional relationship that if X occurs then Y follows (i.e., cause-effect relationship);

4. Be Consistent

If a client engages in an inappropriate behavior that is consequenced inconsistently, it will take longer for the behavior to decrease. *Behavior Contract* may occur when an inappropriate behavior comes under stimulus control, it may be reduced under certain conditions but increased when consequences do not follow; and,

5. Communicate the "Rules of the Game"

When implementing programs to decrease behaviors, the specific behaviors that are to be de-

Adapted from Bernstein et al., *Behavioral Habilitation through Proactive Programming.* Copyright © 1981 by Paul H. Brookes Publishing Co., Inc. Baltimore. Used by permission.

creased should be clearly communicated to the client. Posting the rules is helpful, particularly when using response-cost programs. Clear communication of the rules helps to establish the functional relationship between behavior and its consequences.

MODULE IV—HANDOUT #1
REINFORCER QUESTIONNAIRE

(see Bernstein et al. 1981, p. 159)

Name: _____

Date: _____

Program _____

1. My favorite person is_____

   Things I like to do with him/her are _____

2. The best reward anybody can give me is _____

3. My favorite job at work (or in the unit/group home) is _____

4. If I had $10, I'd _____

5. My favorite relative is _____

6. For a job I want to be _____

7. The person I dislike most is _____

8. Two things I like to do best are _____

9. My favorite staff person is _____

10. When I do something well, the staff _____

11. I feel terrific when _____

12. The way I get money is _____

13. When I have money, I like to _____

14. When I'm in trouble, I_____

15. Something I really want is _____

16. If I had a chance, I sure would like to _____

Adapted from Bernstein et al., *Behavioral Habilitation through Proactive Programming.* Copyright © 1981 by Paul H. Brookes Publishing Co., Inc. Baltimore. Used by permission.

17. The person I like most to reward me is _____

    How?_____

18. I really hate to _____

19. The thing I like to do best with my mother (father) is _____

    _____

20. The thing I do that bothers staff most is_____

21. The weekend activity or entertainment I enjoy most is _____

22. If I did better work, I wish my instructors would _____

23. The kind of punishment I dislike the most is _____

24. My favorite food is _____

25. It sure makes me angry when I can't _____

26. My favorite sport is _____

27. My favorite brother or sister is_____

28. The thing I like to do most is _____

29. The only person I will take advice from is_____

30. My favorite TV programs are_____

MODULE IV—HANDOUT #2
POSSIBLE REINFORCERS

◇◇◇

(see Bernstein et al. 1981, p. 161)

Food
Hot chocolate; popcorn; peanuts; raisins; juices; cookies; donuts; fruit;

A Positive Approach
Patting shoulder; shaking hands; leaning over; eating with; standing alongside; touching arm; touching hand; squeezing hand; helping put on coat; talking with; sitting near; walking alongside;

Expression of Approval
Looking; smiling; grinning; signaling OK; laughing; shrugging shoulders; nodding; cheering; raising eyebrows; slowly closing eyes; chuckling; thumbs up;

Words and Written Symbols of Approval
Fine; OK; well done; wow; good; very good; great; A-1; good work; nicely done; excellent; outstanding; congratulations;

Things
Tokens; surprise packages; paycheck; money; pictures; magazines; newspaper; radio; television movie.

Individual Activities and Privileges
Free time; choosing activities; helping others; leading discussions; displaying work;

Social
Movies; playing music; field trips; planning daily activities; participating in group activities; reading;

Playthings
Athletic equipment; puzzles; commercial games; computer activities;

Reinforcers That May be Used on the Unit or in the Group Home
Choosing a particular food menu; watching a movie; chores; sleeping in on the weekend; going on errands; going out to a special restaurant; taking pictures of friends;

Reinforcers That May Be Used in the Workshop
Time alone with another client; going out to lunch; working on a special task; building a personal project; learning to operate a new tool/machinery; variation in completing daily/weekly tasks; time alone with a staff member.

MODULE IV—HANDOUT # 3
BEHAVIOR TRACKING DAY-TO DAY, WEEK-TO-WEEK, QUANTIFIABLE EVALUATION MEASURES CODING SHEET

The author gratefully acknowledges the information for the "Coding Sheet" developed by Iverson, G.I., & Hughes, R. (2000) Monitoring Aggression and Problem Behaviors in Inpatient Neuropsychiatric Units. *Psychiatric Service* 51, 1040- 1042.

Aggressive Behavior (AB)
1. Threat (physical or verbal)
2. Grabbing
3. Pushing
4. Hitting/kicking
5. Throwing objects
6. Sexually inappropriate
7. Spitting or biting

Other Behavior (OB) or Incident
1. Yelling
2. Verbally abusive/swearing
3. Agitated
4. Pacing/running
5. Interfering/Intrusive
6. Demanding
7. Uncooperative or resistive
8. Angry or hostile
9. Stealing
10. Self-injury or threat to self-injury
11. Damaging Property
12. Medication refusal/medical procedure refusal
13. Refusing to eat
14. Refusing program/activities
15. Refusing home visit
16. Elopement
17. Attempting to leave Unit/group home
18. Substance use/abuse
19. To promote sleep
20. Disruptive
21. Tearful/crying
22. Pre-sedation
23. Paranoid, fearful
24. Smoking violation
25. Hallucinations
26. Delusions

Antecedents / Triggers (A)

1. None/Not observed
2. Noisy Environment
3. Invasion of personal space or invading personal space of others
4. Argument
5. Threatened by co-patient
6. Assaulted by co-patient
7. Verbally teased or antagonized
8. Staff providing personal care
9. Staff setting limits or enforcing rules
10. Delusional or hallucinating
11. Confused state
12. Demanding cigarettes or soft drinks
13. Excessive fluid intake
14. Family visit

PRN Effect (PRN)

1. No effect
2. Moderate – some effect (more settled)
3. Good - settled

Participants (P)

1. Patients only (pt. to pt.)
2. Staff only (pt. to staff)
3. Patients and staff

Injuries (I)

1. To a co-patient
2. To staff
3. To the original patient

Seclusion/Time-out (sec.)

In hour and minutes

Consequences (C)

1. Separation
2. PRN
3. Seclusion
4. Time – Out
5. Mechanical restraint
6. Brief Counseling
7. Re-directed
8. Grounds Withheld
9. Fluid Restriction OT/RT

Location (L)

1. Dayroom
2. Smoking Room
3. Dormitory
4. Washroom
5. Tub Room
6. Hallway
7. Dining Room
8. Around Nursing Office
9. OT/RT
10. Grounds
11. Penn Hall
12. Airing Court
13. Multipurpose Room
14. Elevator
15. Around the Exit Door
16. On Visit Leave

Problem Behavior Recording System – Recording Sheet (Example)

Resident Name:_____ Unit _____

Date Time: AB OB A P I C PRN Sec L

0730
1130
1530
1930
0730
1130
1530
1930
0730
1130
1530
1930
0730
1130
1530
1930

For example, Criteria for behavioral token *reward zero* tolerance for: _____

Refuse token if: _____

AB

OB 2, 10, 11, 18

Sec.

MODULE V

Maintenance and Generalization of Behavior Change
(see Bernstein et al. 1981, Chapter 11)

Concept

1. Maintenance and generalization of positive behavior changes are necessary in order for their changes to be meaningful;

2. Maintenance—more specifically "response maintenance"—refers to continued occurrence of a behavior over time;

3. Generalization is referred to as "stimulus generalization." The occurrence of a behavior under stimulus conditions that are different in some way from the conditions in which the behavior was trained (e.g., hospital inpatients learning appropriate coping strategies that generalize when the patients are discharged to a group home).

TECHNIQUES FOR PROMOTING MAINTENANCE AND GENERALIZATION
TECHNIQUES INVOLVING ANTECEDENTS

Generalization has two different levels:

(a) Behavior will occur under a variety of different conditions within a training program (e.g., compliance to occur in the presence of a variety of different staff);

(b) Generalization from the training program to the natural environment (e.g., behaviors that have been trained on unit to generalize from the training situation to a regular job or community group home situation).

Varying Training Conditions
It is necessary to teach clients to perform behaviors in many different examples of the conditions under which these behaviors have to occur (e.g., noise level, time of day, wording of instructions given).

Equate Stimulus Conditions with the Natural Environment
Make the training conditions as much like the natural environment as possible. The more the training situation is like the natural situation, the more likely it is that the behavior that was learned in the training situation will generalize.

Use of Consequences
Naturally occurring reinforcers are rewards for behaviors that occur in the environments where you want the behavior to occur.

Adapted from Bernstein et al., *Behavioral Habilitation through Proactive Programming.* Copyright © 1981 by Paul H. Brookes Publishing Co., Inc. Baltimore. Used by permission.

Three cautions you need to keep in mind:

(a) A reinforcer is only a reinforcer for a specific client if it increases that individual's behavior (i.e., don't assume a particular consequence maintains everyone's behavior);

(b) There is no single natural environment; there are many natural environments. Make sure that the naturally occurring reinforcers you choose really do occur in the client's relevant environments; and,

(c) You may wish to pair consequences that you would like to become reinforcing for a particular client with consequences that are already reinforcing for that person (e.g., one natural consequence that is often paired with existing reinforcers is *verbal praise*).

"Thin" Schedules of Reinforcement

Behavior is more likely to persist under intermittent reinforcement conditions. In order to achieve behavior that is maintained on a "thin" intermittent schedule of reinforcement, you will need to plan to gradually reduce the amount, frequency and consistency of reinforcement over time. If you start to thin a schedule of reinforcement and the behavior you are interested in maintaining begins to drop off, that usually means reinforcement is being removed too quickly. The clinical staff needs to back up and thin the schedule more gradually. Ideally the end goal should be to have the behavior maintained on a schedule that is as much as possible like the schedule that occurs in the natural environment.

Increase Delays in Reinforcement

In order to increase the likelihood that behavior will continue to occur at a desired level after a move to the natural environment (e.g., group home) you need to see that behavior is reinforced somewhat more frequently in the new environment than it has been in the training environment (e.g., hospital unit).

Two ways to complete this include:

(a) Add new reinforcers to the natural environment and then gradually fade them out to help support the behavior during the initial transition; and

(b) Gradually reduce the frequency and consistency of reinforcement in the training program until the client is receiving less reinforcement than what the natural environment will provide. Then, when the move is made to the natural environment, the amount of reinforcement for the desired behavior will be greater than what it has been in the training setting.

Teach Self-Management to clients diagnosed with psychogenic polydipsia

Self-management of both antecedents and consequences should be taught at some point (*i.e.*, symptoms in the mild range of psychogenic polydipsia) to foster management of the client's own behavior by that client.

(a) Self-Management of Antecedents

Managing antecedents involves altering stimuli that happen just before behavior is to occur. Three ways to complete this are as follows:

i. Clients tell themselves what to do;

ii. Clients arrange cues in their environment that remind them what to do; and

iii. Others (e.g., staff) are asked by the client to provide cues.

(b) Self-Management of Consequences

Self-management of consequences is management of what occurs after a behavior. It has four parts:

i. Self-reporting of behavior;

ii. Self-evaluation of behavior;

iii. Self-determination of consequences; and

iv. Self-administration of those consequences

The development of self-management skills is a gradual process like the learning of any new behavior and must be initially supported by outside consequences like any other behavior.

The first stage in developing self-management skills with regard to consequences is developing the skills to record the client's behavior.

The second stage is the development of skills in evaluating the client's behavior. The inpatients on a closed (i.e., locked) hospital unit often have not learned how to evaluate their own behavior. They frequently do not know how to tell when they have done a good job on a particular task. Standards should be set by the clinical staff to help the client with psychogenic polydipsia decide when a behavior is acceptable and when it is not.

The third stage of self-management of consequences is learning to decide what the appropriate consequence is for a particular behavior. To do this you have to know what consequences you have under control and are therefore able to deliver. One area the clients have control of is how they use their time. The final stage in learning to self-manage consequences is successfully delivering personal reinforcements when the individual has earned it.

A SYSTEMATIC PROGRAMMING STRATEGY

There is a core set of behaviors common to all behavioral approaches:

Adapted from Bernstein et al., *Behavioral Habilitation through Proactive Programming*. Copyright © 1981 by Paul H. Brookes Publishing Co., Inc. Baltimore. Used by permission.

1. A strong commitment to the data-based evaluation of intervention procedures;

2. A belief that staff intervention must include opportunities tolerance of adaptive behavior;

3. The specification of interventions in operational terms; and

4. The evaluation of intervention effects across various response measures with particular emphasis on overt observable behavior.

A Systems approach to behavior

This approach implies that you must view the working shift with residents as composed of behavioral systems and subsystems that function as a whole. They also function as a whole by virtue of the interdependence of their parts. No single behavior or group of behaviors exists in isolation. Program strategy consists of the following steps:

1. Define the problem;

2. Describe what you think is maintaining the problem;

3. Identify possible program options that will solve the problems;

4. Choose from among those options;

5. Evaluate the results of the options selected;

6. (a) If the program is effective, program for maintenance and generalization of the behavioral change; or,

   (b) If the program is not effective, try to figure out why not and change the program so that it will be effective

   (see flow chart below);

A FLOW CHART FOR PROGRAM STRATEGY

(see Bernstein et al. 1981, p. 218)

DEFINE THE CLIENT PROBLEM

FORMULATE HYPOTHESES—WHY

IDENTIFY PROGRAM OPTIONS

SELECT A PROGRAM THAT IS "DOABLE"

EVALUATE THE PROGRAM RESULTS (E.G., BASELINE/TREATMENT)

NOT EFFECTIVE

(REVISE)

*EFFECTIVE

*PROGRAM FOR MAINTENANCE AND GENERALIZATION

CLASSIFICATION SYSTEM FOR BEHAVIOR EXCESSES OR DEFICITS

(see Bernstein et al. 1981, p. 224)

Classifying the type of behavior problem helps staff to think about how the problem might be solved. A classification system divides behavior problems into two general categories: deficits and excesses.

Possible Correlates of Behavior Excess/Deficits:
1. Target behavior is not in the client's repertoire;

2. Antecedent events difficulties:

   a) Relevant areas are too restricted in number or type;

   b) Relevant area is not available.

   Irrelevant areas interfere with recognition of relevant areas:

   a) Emotional arousal interferes with recognition of relevant areas;

   b) Inappropriate cues available in the environment;

   c) Occurrence of internal cues for inappropriate behavior;

   d) Training cue not sufficiently similar to naturally occurring cues.

3. Consequence Difficulties:

   Environment not sufficiently reinforcing

Adapted from Bernstein et al., *Behavioral Habilitation through Proactive Programming*. Copyright © 1981 by Paul H. Brookes Publishing Co., Inc. Baltimore. Used by permission.

a) Source of reinforcement unreliable;

b) Schedule inadequate;

c) Too few sources of reinforcement externally or internally.

Competing behavior reinforcers

a) Naturally occurring reinforcers are more powerful than those available from the training environment; and

b) Self-reinforcement of competing behavior.

4. Inappropriate use of punishment:

a) Too many or too severe aversive consequences relative to availability;

b) Inappropriate self-punishment; and

c) The client does not have acceptable alternative behavior in his or her repertoire.

MODULE VI
Evaluation and Adaptation Procedures
(see Bernstein et al., 1981, pp. 249 – 251)

Checklist for Evaluating Each Client's IPC

EVALUATION ITEM   **SCORING**

A. Match the Curriculum to the Client Need

1.	Do the goals of the IPC meet the client's needs as indicated by their LTG's and STG's?	YES	NO

B. Skills of the Client

1.	Does the IPC have specifically stated LTG's?	YES	NO
2.	Does the IPC specifically state STG's?	YES	NO
3.	Are the STG's analyzed within the overall IPC?	YES	NO
4.	Within the IPC, do the STG's provide functional task analysis of the LTG's?	YES	NO

Does the IPC make provisions for assessing the client's skills across the relevant domains? (Assessment of baseline data).

5.	Are specific prerequisite skills for each STG stated?	YES	NO
6.	Does baseline information result in identification of deficits in behavior?	YES	NO

C. Structure of IPC

1.	Are specific implementation procedures stated?	YES	NO
2.	Are the directions for teaching the skills/concepts understandable to you?	YES	NO
3.	Are the STG's stated in a hierarchy from simple to complex (sequenced)?	YES	NO
4.	Are the STG's dependent or independent of each other (can goals be extracted from the IPC and utilized independently, or are they prerequisites for each other)?	YES	NO
5.	Is the IPC developed to ensure short learning tasks, frequent renewal and frequent testing?	YES	NO

D. Data Collection and Program Assessment

1.	Are techniques for measurement of client progress specifically stated?	YES	NO
2.	Are measurement procedures clear and understandable to you (e.g., are specific behaviors for meeting criteria stated operationally)?	YES	NO

E. Maintenance of Acquired Skills

1.	Does the IPC provide for periodic monitoring of acquired skills on a regular basis? (e.g., at least weekly)?	YES	NO
2.	A review of acquired skills?	YES	NO
3.	Are specific criteria stated for re-entry into the training program?	YES	NO

Adapted from Bernstein et al., *Behavioral Habilitation through Proactive Programming*. Copyright © 1981 by Paul H. Brookes Publishing Co., Inc. Baltimore. Used by permission.

4.	Does the IPC specify what training should follow the acquisition of a skill?	**YES**	**NO**
5.	Are criteria for termination of the maintenance portion of the IPC specified?	**YES**	**NO**

F. Validation of the IPC

1.	Was the IPC field-tested (e.g., baseline, treatment)?	**YES**	**NO**
2.	Are the client characteristics identified (e.g., age, sex, disabilities, capabilities)?	**YES**	**NO**
3.	Are the characteristics of the training setting identified (e.g., resource room etc.,)?	**YES**	**NO**

G. Practical Considerations

1.	Budgetary requirements?	**YES**	**NO**
2.	Are the directions for teaching the skills/concepts understandable to you?	**YES**	**NO**
3.	Is the teaching mode of the IPC specified in terms of needed requirements of doing the program?	**YES**	**NO**
4.	Do you have the physical facilities to accommodate the IPC program?	**YES**	**NO**
5.	Is the amount of time (per day or week) that must be devoted to the IPC specified?	**YES**	**NO**
6.	Is the staff/client ratio for effective implementation specified?	**YES**	**NO**

Adapted from Bernstein et al., *Behavioral Habilitation through Proactive Programming*. Copyright © 1981 by Paul H. Brookes Publishing Co., Inc. Baltimore. Used by permission.

MODULE VI— HANDOUT #1
WORKSHEET FOR BEHAVIOR PROBLEM ANALYSIS

(see Bernstein et al. 1981, p. 219)

Resident: _____

Date: _____ Staff Completing the Analysis: _____

EVALUATION OF PROBLEM	POSSIBLE CORRELATES	OPTIONS
DOES DO / SHOULD DO CLASSIFICATION	PROG. (GOAL)	RESOURCES OPTIONS +'S -'S

MODULE VI— HANDOUT # 2
PROGRAM FORM

◇◇◇

(see Bernstein et al., 1981, p. 233)

Resident: _____

Date Program Begins: _____

I. Behavior
a) Target Behavior _____

b) Current Behavior _____

c) Why the program is needed _____

II. Conditions
a) Where? (location) _____

b) When? (schedule) _____

c) With what? (material) _____

d) By whom? (people responsible) _____

III. Method
What to do and how to do it?

1. Before behavior occurs (antecedents) _____

2. After behavior occurs (consequences and contingencies) _____

_____

_____

IV. Evaluation
a) Attach completed Measurement Procedure Form

b) Who is responsible for regular review of the data? _____

c) When are these reviews to occur?_____

PRE/POST QUIZ
CULTURE CHANGE IN THE WORK ENVIRONMENT

To be administered prior to Module I and after Module VI

1. Change that is mandated is:
   a) Less often
   b) Often
   c) More often likely to occur

2. Focus your efforts on supporting desired behaviors rather than on eliminating unwanted behaviors is:
   a) Sometimes appropriate
   b) Appropriate
   c) Sometimes inappropriate
   d) Inappropriate

3. What is the purpose of the development of the IPC?
   a) Change undesired behavior as identified by nursing staff and other professionals
   b) Evaluate the program
   c) Improve communication
   d) A, B and C

4. When evaluating goals, what will be taken into consideration?
   a) Time and frequency
   b) Rate and accuracy
   c) A and B
   d) A but not B

5. What are operationalized terms?

   a) Outcome of the goal
   b) Observable and measurable descriptions of behavior
   c) Resident's behaviors
   d) Outcomes of the IPC

6. Direction of change refers to what is to be accomplished with the individual's behavior.
   a) True
   b) False

7. What are two ways to approach behavioral problems?
   a) Implement programs designed to decrease behavior
   b) Implement programs to increase the period of time between undesired behaviors
   c) Both of the above
   d) None of the above

8. When defining residents' behavior in specific or operational terms, you need to use observable and measurable terms.
   a) Sometimes true
   b) True
   c) False
   d) Sometimes false

9. What are the five dimensions of behavior?
   a) Realistic, understandable, measurable, positive, behaviors
   b) Frequency, duration, latency, form, intensity

10. When is true sampling used?
   a) For infrequent behaviors
   b) For frequent behaviors

11. A.B.C. model of behavior provides us with:
   a) Description of events
   b) Description of behavior and events
   c) Events before the behavior and events that follow a behavior
   d) None of the above

12. PREMACK principle refers to:
   a) High probability behavior that could be used as reward for low probability behavior.
   b) Maladaptive behavior reinforces adaptive behavior
   c) Both A and B
   d) Sometimes A but not B

13. Reinforcement is defined as:
   a) Its conditioning effect
   b) Its effect on behavior
   c) Neither of the above
   d) A and B

14. Variable reinforcement is:
   a) More reinforcing than intermittent reinforcement
   b) Maintains a behavior for long periods of time without reinforcement
   c) More resistant to the loss of reinforcement
   d) B and C

15. Differential reinforcement of other behavior (DRO) is:
  a) Never delivered when the patient is fatigued
  b) Delivered on a schedule for the nonoccurrence of a target behavior
  c) None of the above
  d) A and B

16. Extinction procedures are effective when:
  a) Combined with positive reinforcement procedures
  b) Reinforcement is no longer presented
  c) A and B
  d) None of the above

17. Maintenance and generalization are:
  a) Absolutely necessary in order for patient change to be meaningful
  b) Happens in a "lock step" fashion
  c) Only occurs when implemented in combination with "thinning" procedures
  d) A and C

18. Teaching self-management occurs when:
  a) The resident tells him/herself what to do
  b) The resident arranges cues in his/her environment that are reminders of what to do
  c) Others (e.g., staff, family) are asked by the residents to provide cues
  d) All of the above

19. The development of self-management skills are:
  a) Quickly learned through reinforcement techniques/consequences
  b) A gradual process (two steps forward, one step backward)
  c) A and B
  d) None of the above

20. Systematic programming strategy involves:
  a) A strong commitment to data-based evaluation
  b) Adaptive behaviors that are learned
  c) Interventions by staff that are operationalized terms
  d) All of the above

QUIZ ANSWERS

Culture Change in the Work Environment

1-a, 2-b, 3-d, 4-c, 5-b, 6-a, 7-c, 8-b, 9-b, 10-b, 11-c, 12-a, 13-b, 14-d, 15-b, 16-c, 17-d, 18-d, 19-b , 20-d

CHAPTER FOUR

PSYCHOSOCIAL REHABILITATION AS IT PERTAINS TO PSYCHOGENIC POLYDIPSIA

Concepts

The following information is taken from the psychosocial rehabilitation/readaptation (PSR/RPS) Canadian Code of Ethics (2010). These principles and values are related to evidence-based PSR practices and informed by the lived experiences of individuals with mental health challenges.

Psychosocial rehabilitation (PSR) promotes personal recovery, successful community integration, and satisfactory quality of life for persons who have a mental illness or mental health concerns. Psychosocial rehabilitation services and supports are collaborative, person-directed, and individualized, and they are an essential element of the treatment paradigm for clients diagnosed with psychogenic polydipsia. They focus on clients developing skills and access to resources needed to increase their capacity to be successful and satisfied in a myriad of living, learning and working environments.

PSR/RPS CORE PRINCIPLES AND VALUES

1. Psychosocial rehabilitation practitioners convey hope and respect, and they believe that all individuals have the capacity for learning and growth;

2. Psychosocial rehabilitation practitioners recognize that culture and diversity are central to recovery, and they strive to ensure that all services and supports are culturally relevant to individuals receiving services and supports;

3. Psychosocial rehabilitation practitioners engage in the processes of informed and shared decision-making and facilitate partnerships with other persons identified by the individual receiving services and supports;

4. Psychosocial rehabilitation practices build on strengths and capacities of individuals receiving services and supports;

5. Psychosocial rehabilitation practices are person-centered; they are designed to address the distinct needs of individuals, consistent with their values, hopes and aspirations;

6. Psychosocial rehabilitation practices support full integration of people in recovery into their communities, where they can exercise their rights of citizenship, accept the responsibilities, and explore the opportunities that come with being a member of a community and a larger society;

7. Psychosocial rehabilitation practices promote self-determination and empowerment. All individuals have the right to make their own decisions, including decisions about the types of services and supports they receive;

8. Psychosocial rehabilitation practices facilitate the development of personal support networks by utilizing natural supports within communities, family members as defined by the individual, peer support initiatives, and self- and mutual-help groups;

9. Psychosocial rehabilitation practices strive to help individuals improve the quality of all aspects of their lives, including social, occupational, educational, residential, intellectual, spiritual, and financial;

10. Psychosocial rehabilitation practices promote health and wellness and encourage individuals to develop and use individualized wellness plans;

11. Psychosocial rehabilitation services and supports emphasize evidence-based, promising, and emerging best practices that produce outcomes congruent with personal recovery. Psychosocial rehabilitation programs include program evaluation and continuous quality improvement that actively involve persons receiving services and supports;

12. Psychosocial rehabilitation services and supports must be readily accessible to all individuals whenever they need them; these services and supports should be well coordinated and integrated as needed with other psychiatric, medical, and holistic treatments and practices.

PRINCIPLES OF EFFECTIVE PSYCHOSOCIAL TREATMENT FOR SCHIZOPHRENIA

The principles articulated below have emerged from disparate studies and represent a convergence of clinical and research endeavors.

As a general statement, psychosocial interventions based on social learning principles, therapeutic community, and educational methods, need to be applied in a 24-hour, highly structured, consistent, and socially engineered environment. Targeted symptoms regarding clients diagnosed with psychogenic polydipsia are primarily deviant behavior that impedes adjustment in less restrictive environments (i.e., residential group homes in the community). Interventions should be directed at reducing behavioral deviances (e.g., excesses of maladaptive behavior) as well as strengthening adaptive abilities that will compensate for the resident's deficits. Social-skills training has been shown to be particularly valuable as a treatment modality. Interventions need to be designed to engage the schizophrenic client diagnosed with psychogenic polydipsia, whose positive symptoms (e.g., thought disorder, distractibility) are exacerbated by excessive fluid ingestion.

Teaching attention and learning capabilities with this clinical population requires highly trained staff who can develop a positive working relationship with the clients. This often requires strategic and paradoxical interventions as well as a stable therapeutic team capable of engaging clients in a positive relationship with rapport, patience, and professionalism.

Co-occurrent disordered, schizophrenic clients diagnosed with psychogenic polydipsia have long standing, over-learned symptoms and behavioral deficits / excesses that yield slowly to changed environmental contingencies. Improvement may occur only after many years of sustained and consistent treatment. The major issue is aimed at small, gradual, and incremental goals, with progress of any magnitude matched by abundant positive reinforcement from the multidisciplinary team. Clients diagnosed with psychogenic polydipsia should be involved as much as possible in the selection, sequencing, and prioritizing of psychosocial treatment goals and the monitoring and reinforcement of progress. This requires the clinical team to educate the client about the nature of his or her illness (e.g., schizophrenia and psychogenic polydipsia) and the reality of real change occurring (i.e., "two steps forward one back").

Durability and generalization of treatment effects require planned orchestration of the therapeutic interventions. The multidisciplinary team should promote and reinforce any therapeutic change, conducting at least a portion of the daily treatment in the client's continuum of care options in the community. The transfer of treatment effects from an inpatient hospital environment to a community residential living arrangement is augmented if the client's relatives and caregivers are involved with the therapeutic process from the outset. Gradual "fading" of the intensity and structure of the psychosocial therapy should be an established priority in the current inpatient environment, by using more intermittent sessions and reinforcement strategies and then blending these techniques with the client's discharge to a reduced level of community care.

A centralized, organizational hierarchy is a primary obstacle to becoming a rehab-ready community facility for clients diagnosed with psychogenic polydipsia. This administration model that is seen in the hospital structure should be replaced with a decentralized, interdisciplinary rehabilitation model for psychosocial treatment initiatives with this clinical population. More specifically, a team leader (i.e., group home supervisor) should be given final decision-making authority on treatment schedules and direct-care staff responsibilities. Thus with primary supervisory responsibility and authority over the psychosocial treatment team (e.g., paraprofessional staff, social worker, psychologist, occupational therapist, recreation staff, nursing staff, dietician) the team leader is able to better integrate staff into the treatment team and make any scheduling adjustments necessary to meet the needs of the program.

In conjunction, direct performance-based feedback is possible, which is often not the case with a centralized model in which supervisors can be far removed from the actual treatment setting. Finally, team leaders can take disciplinary action as needed.

Psychosocial treatment of clients diagnosed with psychogenic polydipsia is designed to meet the rehabilitation needs of dual diagnosed, severely mentally ill residents with multiple skill deficits. These individuals require extended inpatient care prior to discharge to a "step-down" structured community living environment. Psychosocial treatment paradigms are an integrated network of learning-based techniques and skills-training technologies comprehensively applied by the clinical staff, across the waking hours of the clients, for all problem areas. Emphasis is placed on decreasing bizarre, unusual, and aggressive behaviors and on improving self-care skills, problem solving, social skills, and vocational and leisure-time skills.

A core tenet of psychosocial treatment programs is that all interactions between staff and clients have the potential to be therapeutic. Staff is expected to deliver high rates of verbal and nonverbal praise in response to appropriate client behavior, thus reinforcing these behaviors and encouraging their continued occurrence. Development of new adaptive behaviors is accomplished through modeling and direct instruction.

Shaping procedures are a very important ingredient of psychosocial treatment programs and are essential to teaching behaviors and skills to clients diagnosed with psychogenic polydipsia. This consists of breaking down a behavior into smaller component behaviors and reinforcing successive approximations.

Target behaviors are made progressively more difficult by increasing the amount of time that must be spent on the task by increasing the complexity of the task. Reinforcement consists of verbal and nonverbal praise, snacks, and tokens that can be redeemed in the treatment setting for a variety of consumables or privileges. The skills that are targeted by the psychosocial treatment programs include "on-task" participation in groups, appropriate social interaction, self-care (hygiene) activities, and challenging and replacing "automatic thoughts" about seeking and overdrinking fluids with more appropriate activities. Psychosocial treatment is also designed to decrease maladaptive behaviors and substitute more appropriate and adaptive behaviors. Substantial effort is directed toward assuring that clients receive attention for appropriate and adaptive behaviors and not for maladaptive behaviors.

A further concern expressed by service providers is that the addition of effective psychosocial strategies to optimal medication trials requires more professional time than is presently available in community-based services for this particular clinical population.

Researchers have shown that, over the course of a year, substantial professional time is saved when effective strategies are used (Held, 1995; Brooker, Falloon, Butterworth, Goldberg, Graham-Hole, & Hillier, 1994). Most of the reduction in time results from reductions in crisis management and hospital care. In services where hospital and community units function independently, the savings from one may come at the expense of the other. In a field trial with community nurses, Brooker and colleagues (1994) showed that the weekly time spent per identified respondent was 33 minutes for the nonspecific treatment approach and 47 minutes for the comprehensive psychosocial approach. The latter resulted in a tenfold reduction in time spent in hospital! The implications of using skilled community resources are clear and would appear to answer many of the current concerns about improving mental health services while containing costs. There can, in the author's opinion, be no reasonable justification for not implementing effective and efficient psychosocial mental health strategies for those clients diagnosed with psychogenic polydipsia. The only problem for services is to choose the precise approach to implement, provide training for all staff, and review the quality of application of the methods to improve and maintain competence.

In this regard, multidisciplinary teams, delivering integrated hospital and community services, should be trained to administer effective treatment strategies in an adept manner with this complex, hard-to-treat clinical population (i.e., co-occurrent disorder). More specifically, the needs are:

- Continuous audits on at least a quarterly basis of the program's quality and supervisory skills;

- Independent standards of the clinical, social, and economic benefits of the psychosocial treatment program;

- Workbooks and manuals to enhance the consistency of treatment for this clinical population. They should be developed with continuous reviews conducted to examine the fidelity of applications of the psychosocial strategies and to provide continuing enhancement of the clinical skills of the treatment team; and

- A set of outcome measures that can be applied in clinical practice, devised from existing "global scales" (e.g., Brief Psychiatric Rating Scale).

Continuity of care is critical to assist clients diagnosed with psychogenic polydipsia, maintaining and building upon the gains made in the psychosocial treatment programs as inpatients in a hospital setting.

This clientele are, with time, usually discharged to a step-down hospital unit (i.e., open unit, not secured), which is followed, by discharge to a community-based group home rehabilitation cottage. Thus, as the more severely afflicted and aggressive SIWI residents improve within the locked, hospital unit, learning more effective ways to control aggressive impulses and tendencies, they are transferred to less restrictive living arrangements where they continue to develop skills-training opportunities. The opportunity to be discharged to a continuum of community-based rehabilitation cottages, with staff trained to deal effectively with psychogenic polydipsia, increases the potential of successful transfers from the inpatient hospital programs. The community programs and their linkage to the hospital inpatient programs for this clinical population is generally more tolerant of risk (due in part to staff training and expertise) yet affords more rehabilitation opportunities and privileges than are available in the hospital milieu. Clients diagnosed with psychogenic polydipsia who are living in the community group home system receive a continuum of care that allows for each person to maximize skill level and self-sufficiency. In such instances, the linkage between the hospital inpatient units servicing this clientele assist the staff in the community group homes in developing a continuity of care, Individual Program Plans (IPP) that will capitalize on gains made and provide consultation privileges to community providers.

PSYCHOLOGICAL RISK FACTORS PRECIPITATED BY PSYCHOGENIC POLYDIPSIA

Overconsumption of any/all fluids during a 24-hour period with clients diagnosed with psychogenic polydipsia can precipitate self-induced water intoxication (SIWI). During the state of intoxication, the SIWI client's aberrant behavioral repertoire can include self-initiated exposure to conditions such as walking on busy roadways, entering private homes or property without permission and at unacceptable times, elopement from supervised settings, physical aggression, property destruction, and threats of violence, sexual assault, and self-injury. The risk factor for repeated occurrence of this maladaptive behavior while the individual is in a state of fluid intoxication includes the following features of personal vulnerability (Gardner & Hunter, 2003):

1. Deficits in skills of self-monitoring and self-modulation of heightened arousal such as anger, irritability, or inappropriate sexual arousal;

2. Deficits in skills to self-regulate (monitor and inhibit) impulsive acts, (i.e., poor impulse control skills);

3. Deficits in skills of communication, problem solving, and interpersonal conflict resolution skills, as well as deficits in prosocial skill and social competencies as alternatives to interpersonal and personal conflict;

4. Deficits in skills of self-selecting and initiating alternative prosocial coping strategies;

5. Deficits in a socialized motivational system that values prosocial alternatives. More specifically, deficits in empathic skills to cognitively and emotionally anticipate the effects on others of impulsive acts such as physical or sexual aggression, property destruction, threats of violence, reduced social motivation to please others or assist others, and to adhere to socially appropriate standards of conduct;

6. Deficits in social motivation involving concern over creating distress in others;

7. Deficits in social motivation to develop positive affective attachments with others; and,

8. Deficits in the motivational bias for assuming personal responsibility for one's behavior. This includes deficits in the cognitive and emotional internalization of socially appropriate standards of conduct. SIWI clients are thus without effective internalized standards against which to judge the appropriateness of their behaviors or to be motivated to self-regulate them.

To emphasize the *Psychosocial Treatment Model* for clients with episodic SIWI, it is imperative that the treatment model is individually designed to address the array of psychological, social, physical, environmental, medical, psychiatric, and neuropsychiatric conditions identified. This is achieved through appropriate diagnostic assessments that evaluate each client's behavioral and related psychiatric symptoms that resulted in hospital placement.

SIWI TREATMENT VS. STABILIZATION

It should be noted that effective treatment of the personal (medical, psychiatric, and behavioral) conditions resulting in the dangerous behavioral symptoms differs from a process of stabilization of these behavioral symptoms following hospital placement. A client diagnosed with psychogenic polydipsia who is SIWI and manifesting dangerous symptoms may abate following a period of stabilization and removal from the crisis-producing conditions (e.g., abrasive co-resident). These stressors, as interpreted by the SIWI client, that cause fluid-seeking behavior, over-ingestion, and intoxication often result in rage-producing interpersonal provocations, environmental constraints and other antisocial behavior stated above.

Once the SIWI intoxication has abated, the client's behavioral symptoms become reduced or disappear in the hospital's managed environment. Needless to say, unless the SIWI client's propensity to seek out and overdrink any/all fluids becomes manageable, they will remain vulnerable to recurrence of the behavioral symptoms when exposed to symptom-producing conditions upon entry to a community living environment. That is the therapeutic challenge!

METHODS OF PROVIDING PSYCHOSOCIAL INTERVENTION TO SIWI CLIENTS

Clients diagnosed with psychogenic polydipsia with chronic SIWI require a psychosocial treatment program from a myriad of professional disciplines (e.g., social work, family physician, psychology, psychiatry, dietician, recreation therapy, occupational therapy, and physiotherapy) to enhance assimilation of self-monitoring, self-evaluation, and self-instructional behavior. This combination of skills, paired with exposure to conditions of provocation, leads to eventual practice of the skills *in situ*. The contingent relationship between positive behavior and positive consequences should be rigorously followed throughout the training program. Positive reinforcers are provided frequently and represented concretely by the staff. Progress towards goal attainment is also concretely represented and reviewed frequently. Situations influencing compulsive fluid seeking behavior should be examined by the treatment staff during training. This ensures that SIWI clients can practice counteractive coping strategies/techniques when they are faced with potentially stressful situations in the future. In conjunction, following success in specific situations of provocation, the client is then taught more general problem-solving skills for use in other similar situations.

Specific procedures can include the following coping strategies: thought stopping, counting (visualizing numbers 1-8 to challenge emotional arousal), assertiveness training, diaphragmatic breathing techniques, progressive deep muscle relaxation, self-talk (mantra), and CBT problem-solving skills. All of the above are used to train the residents for generalization of these skills to counter future provocative situations. Of Note: initially train specific coping skills with suitable motivational supports, then teach the individual to self-manage the skills when confronted with problem situations. Subsequently, the client is systematically provided increased independence in decision making relative to behavior-consequence outcomes.

Ideally, the Psychosocial Treatment Model entails increasing the client's triad of interrelated behavioral, emotional, and cognitive competencies. These competencies serve as functional replacements for the need to seek out and overdrink any/all fluids, which place the client at risk for seizure, coma and eventual death. The competencies also replace those personal features mentioned above as being dangerous and disruptive, requiring the SIWI client to remain in a locked, hospital unit thereby reducing the chance for discharge to a less restrictive living environment and enhanced quality of life.

BEHAVIORAL SUPPORTS INTEGRATED AS COMPONENTS OF THE PSYCHOSOCIAL TREATMENT PLAN

The treatment plan for clients diagnosed with psychogenic polydipsia who present recurring behavioral concerns in the hospital or community residential setting, which result in the use of timeout, seclusion, restraints, and PRN's for behavior control, should include: (a) individualized behavioral support strategies and approaches based on comprehensive and integrative biomedical, psychological, social, and physical environmental assessments. The factors influencing occurrence, severity, fluctuation, and durability of these current behavioral concerns; (b) strategies and approaches that are predominately proactive and preventive and specifically designed to avoid undue restraint on the client's freedom of movement; (c) behavioral support strategies and approaches are designed to encourage each client to use prosocial coping skills as alternatives to disruptive actions under the specific antecedent conditions that influence occurrence, severity, and recurrence of the behavioral concerns; (d) the behavior support strategies and approaches are integrated with the client's treatment plan rather than being a separate and independently developed Behavior Support Plan document. The strategies and approaches shall be designed to reduce or eliminate the conditions producing these behavioral concerns, including the development of coping skills to serve as prosocial functional alternatives, rather than merely to manage problematic behavioral symptoms.

THE ASSESSMENT OF PROGRAM EFFECTIVENESS: THE PRESENCE OF AN OBJECTIVE DATA, OBSERVATION, RECORDING, AND TREATMENT EVALUATION SYSTEM

An objective data, observation, recording, and evaluation system should be present to monitor the progress and outcome effectiveness of the separate and combined treatment program components (e.g., behavior and psychosocial sections of the treatment program). Both individualized and program-wide objective data evaluation systems may involve standardized scales and inventories as well as individually developed procedures. These systems support the clinical decision-making process, facilitate a hypothesis-testing approach to case formulation, and provide measures of the impact of interventions. These monitoring systems should be used by the multidisciplinary treatment team to assess the effectiveness of each biomedical and psychosocial intervention and to make timely changes in the treatment approaches when data results dictate.

Each treatment plan, including the behavior support components, should address:

- Specification of staff responsibilities for each component of the plan. Who will do what, when and where will it be done?

- How will implementation be monitored, how and when will program effectiveness be assessed, and who will supervise each component?

- All discharge planning should involve the patient, family, and guardians as appropriate, as well as community service and residential providers.

- A comprehensive matrix of community supports needed for each client should be developed to ensure successful transition and adjustment to community living.

- Specification of responsibilities for delivery and ongoing monitoring of each of the identified community supports should be included in the discharge plan.

Discharge criteria should be objectively defined and reflect consistency with treatment plan objectives and treatment experiences provided in the hospital setting. These criteria should be considered in selection of short- and long-term treatment program objectives.

RELATIONSHIP BETWEEN STAFFING RATIOS AND EFFECTIVENESS OF INPATIENT PSYCHIATRIC UNITS TREATING CLIENTS DIAGNOSED WITH PSYCHOGENIC POLYDIPSIA

Higher staff-client ratios and smaller treatment units have long been identified as the only non-client-related characteristics that are consistently associated with the effectiveness of inpatient units, independent of specific treatment programs (Menditto, 2002). Although these two highly correlated variables lend support to the notion that more staff is better, they account for a small proportion of the variance in any practical measure of inpatient unit effectiveness, such as post-treatment community tenure or discharge rates (Coleman & Paul, 2001). Although staff-client ratios are easy to calculate and readily available, they are, at best, a proxy for the amount of attention that SIWI clients receive from clinical staff. The amount of staff attention varies widely according to staff utilization practices and program structures. Direct observational studies in public mental institutions have shown that clients on a typical unit spend, on average, less than 5% of their waking hours engaged in scheduled therapeutic activities and less than 11% in any contact with staff (Paul, 1986). In one study, differences were observed in the amounts of attention provided by staff to patients across two intramural psychosocial programs that had identical staffing levels (Paul & Lentz, 1977).

Despite equivalent staffing ratios across conditions, clients who were treated in two comprehensive psychosocial programs that demonstrated high rates of staff attention had significantly better community outcomes than clients from comparable hospital programs with lower rates of staff attention. However, the comprehensive program based on social-learning principles remained more effective than the second-best program under conditions of both more and less staff attention. These results indicated that the amount of staff attention that clients received affects unit effectiveness more than staff-client ratios. They also showed that the manner in which staff attention is delivered is even more important in determining unit effectiveness.

Although the literature generally supports the idea that staffing ratios predict unit effectiveness as well as the notion that the amount of attention that clients receive from staff may account for this relationship, findings have not provided answers to two important questions. First, do staff-client ratios explain enough of the variance in practical measures of unit effectiveness to inform staffing decisions? Second, do direct measurement of the amount of staff attention account for the predictive power of staffing ratios, perhaps serving as a better predictor of unit effectiveness than raw staffing ratios? Coleman & Paul's (2001) study answered this question by suggesting that the amount of attention clients receive from staff serves as a better predictor of unit effectiveness than staffing ratios for net gain therapeutically. Staffing ratios were found to account for 24% of the variance in a residualized measure of community tenure, which falls at the midpoint of percentages reported in previous studies that used a variety of unit-effectiveness criteria (Gurel, 1964; Lasky & Dowling, 1971; Linn, 1970; Mapes & Clarke, 1975; Ullmann, 1967). This relatively small magnitude of prediction, combined with the fact that staffing ratios do not predict unit effectiveness when indexed by improvement in discharge rate, indicated that the predictive power of raw staffing ratios is insufficient for making staffing decisions. In addition, the partial correlations showed that staffing ratios are not significantly related to the community tenure measure of unit effectiveness after the amount of staff attention was controlled for. In contrast, the amount of staff attention continued to be significantly associated with both measures of unit effectiveness after staffing ratios were controlled (Coleman et al., 2001).

Direct measurement of the amount of attention that clients receive from staff takes into account both staff utilization and staff activity. Such measurement not only predicts unit effectiveness better than staffing ratios but also explains the observed relationship between staffing ratios and unit effectiveness. Coleman et al's (2001) findings indicated that objective data on the amount of attention clients receive from staff is a more important consideration than staffing ratios in staffing decisions aimed at improving the effectiveness of inpatient treatment programs. Thus it seems that adequate staffing ratios for inpatient SIWI treatment units set the stage for therapeutic interactions.

However, this alone does not guarantee effective treatment. It appears, as mentioned above, a large proportion of staff time and client time, during which therapeutic contacts could occur, is not used for that purpose (Paul, 1986). Coleman's findings indicated that staffing decisions should ensure that desirable amounts of staff attention are provided by means of empirically effective utilization structures and by training direct care staff to use empirically effective intervention techniques (Paul, 2000).

A COMMUNITY-BASED SERVICE SYSTEM AND MODELS OF PSYCHOSOCIAL INTERVENTION FOR CLIENTS DIAGNOSED WITH PSYCHOGENIC POLYDIPSIA

The service system for psychogenic polydipsia during the past five years (i.e., 2006-2011) in British Columbia has been transformed to a substantial yet variable degree. From the only stand-alone provincial psychiatric hospital (Riverview Hospital) to a system of community-based health care centers with fewer inpatient beds and a relatively stronger but still inadequate community-oriented psychiatric system. There are several components of this new model of care, which includes:

- Community mental health or continuing-care teams that provide case management to a subset of clients (i.e., psychogenic polydipsia) with schizophrenia;

- Assertive Community Treatment Teams (ACT) that provide mobile intensive case management to a more complex subset of clients (i.e., psychogenic polydipsia);

- Crisis teams/community assessment and treatment teams that provide acute phase community based assessment and treatment;

- Acute inpatient units in the general hospital setting;

- Subacute inpatient care for treatment-resistant SIWI clients;

- Intensively supervised community-based clinical care residential units for clients diagnosed with psychogenic polydipsia; and

- A range of non-government organization residential and day care facilities.

The effect on practice of this still incomplete wave of reform during this period of time has been initiated as a result of the closure of the only stand-alone psychiatric facility in British Columbia in 2012. Yet very little health-services research has been carried out to assess the impact on clients and families. In this regard, assertive community treatment is strongly supported as a model of care. This style of client-service provision for the clients diagnosed with psychogenic polydipsia provides support for both the crisis/group home treatment model and the intensive, mobile case management (i.e., outreach team) model of intervention. Early intervention models of care for those clients with symptoms of psychogenic polydipsia and continuing-care teams and case management are fundamental building blocks of the system of care, for this difficult clinical population housed in community care facilities. More specifically, assertive case management based on an appropriate skill base from a multidisciplinary team, and moderate case loads to enable flexible outreach, is strongly endorsed for those clients diagnosed with mild/moderate psychogenic polydipsia living in community facilities.

This unique clinical population with a diagnosed co-occurrent disorder requires secure access to specialist multidisciplinary teams familiar with the evidenced-based treatment practices that have been proven effective. The team should also be in partnership with family physicians (G.P's) and community-based psychiatrists. This is done to reduce the problems of quality, resourcing and mutual integration of the various service elements. The problems with clients diagnosed with severe psychogenic polydipsia and treatment refractory schizophrenia is the failure of full remission of positive symptoms or the lack of satisfactory clinical improvement, despite sequential use of recommended doses of two or more antipsychotic medications for 6-8 weeks (McGorry, 2005).

Treatment refractory schizophrenia may be obvious early in the treatment of a client diagnosed with severe psychogenic polydipsia. Compounding the problem is the frequency of overdrinking any/all fluids to a state of self-induced water intoxication (SIWI). The mainstay medication for schizophrenics diagnosed with psychogenic polydipsia has been Clozapine. However, while biological interventions have improved the treatment of many dual diagnosed clients with schizophrenia and psychogenic polydipsia, a majority of these individuals have not made gains in the personal, occupational, social or self-care domains of their lives. In the past 20 years, cognitive interventions have emerged, followed by psycho-education and vocational re-habilitation being developed, which have shown positive results in targeting the symptoms of schizophrenia and psychogenic polydipsia, as well as addressing the wider psychosocial con-sequences. It has been accepted during this period that treatment of schizophrenia and, to a similar degree, psychogenic polydipsia cannot be a one-dimensional biological approach. For optimal outcome, the psychosocial domain needs to be addressed (Huxley, Rendall & Sederer, 2000). The following guidelines have been developed:

- Individuals dually diagnosed with schizophrenia and psychogenic polydipsia should be provided with psychosocial interventions relevant to their needs and informed by an un-derstanding of the social and cultural context by which they are currently living;

- When psychosocial interventions are included in an overall treatment paradigm, quality of life and functioning should be improved in addition to a positive effect on the client's negative symptoms and recovery levels;

- Establishing this type of multilevel care for clients dually diagnosed with schizophrenia and psychogenic polydipsia allows a family a feeling of being more supported and informed and better able to look after their relative during home visits. This treatment approach provides education, rehabilitation, support, and appropriate frequencies of intervention (i.e., 1:1) with the clinical staff, which, if managed properly, has a carry-over generalization effect to the patient's nuclear family;

- Psychosocial interventions work best in a system not totally occupied with managing the acute episodes of illness and then discharging the client to minimalist care (especially where the family physician is the sole clinician) where the potential for relapse will be increased;

- Psychosocial intervention needs to be tailored to the individual and phase of illness (e.g., mild, moderate or severe psychogenic polydipsia) and focus on issues of specific relevance to the respective patients;

- As mentioned many times above, psychosocial interventions require well-trained clinicians with specific expertise! In conjunction, cognitive behavioral therapy (CBT) is effective in reducing symptoms in treatment refractory schizophrenia (Rilling, Bebbington & Kupo-ers, 2002);

- Psycho-education (PE) programs for people dually diagnosed with schizophrenia and psychogenic polydipsia should use the biopsychosocial perspective, especially in the early phase of treatment, which focuses on supporting and educating the client and the family about the illnesses; Psycho-education should be offered as a core intervention;

- Social skills training (SST) improves social adjustment, enlarges and enhances the client's social network and contributes to the development of independent living skills (Kopelow-icz, Liberman & Zarate, 2002); and

- SST improves independent living skills and can generalize to situations outside the inpatient setting. SST in association with longer-term group psychotherapy improves symptoms. SST improves medication and symptom management skills. Activities groups improve social interaction.

RIVERVIEW HOSPITAL PSYCHO-EDUCATIONAL SESSIONS FOR CLIENTS DIAGNOSED WITH PSYCHOGENIC POLYDIPSIA (2003-2006)

Preamble

The Riverview Hospital SIWI Psycho-education Program, many of whose concepts have been discussed in preceding pages, is described in depth below. Budgeting restrictions kept the full therapeutic impact of expanding the program from including other equally important disciplines from becoming directly involved. The author is indebted to Nurse Clinician Jacqui Hlagi B.Sc for developing the program and its final revision in February 2003.

TABLE OF CONTENTS

Psycho-education Program

Introduction

Session I: Self-Induced Water Intoxication (SIWI) – Introductory Session (Nursing)

Part II – Visual Discrimination (Nursing)

Session II: Signs, Symptoms and Impact of SIWI – Quality of Life (Nursing/Physician)

Session III: Healthy Fluid Intake (Part I) (Dietician)

Session IV: Health Fluid Intake (Part II) (Dietician)

Session V: Coping Strategies with SIWI (Psychologist)

SIWI PSYCHO-EDUCATION TEACHING SESSIONS 2003-2006

Introduction

* The purpose of the five rotating sessions is to increase awareness of psychogenic polydipsia and SIWI;

* Encouragement is required for the clients to participate actively in the group. Emphasis on the clients' self-monitoring and taking responsibility for their behavior is the goal of the five sessions;

* Groups may need to be divided into further sessions if needed (e.g., other disciplines join);

* The sessions are to be rotated and held semiweekly in the living milieu of the clients and commence at 8:30 a.m. on Tuesdays and Thursdays;

* Sessions #1 and #2 will be facilitated by nursing staff;

* Sessions #3 and #4 will facilitated by the clinical dietician;

* Session #5 will be facilitated by the psychologist;

* Other members of the multidisciplinary team are welcome to attend the sessions (as guests) to familiarize themselves with the content of the sessions, and various members of the team may also be invited to co-facilitate based on their area of expertise;

* The length of the sessions will be approximately 20 minutes, depending on the attention span of the clients;

* Sessions are held in the conference room of the "water ward" to promote attendance and avoid ward/activity distractions.

SESSION I: PART ONE
SELF - INDUCED WATER INTOXICATION (SIWI)

Definition: What is SIWI?

- Self-induced water intoxication (SIWI) occurs when a client diagnosed with psychogenic polydipsia has a need to overdrink any/all fluids due to increased thirst or excessive fluid intake of greater than 3 L/day;

- The SIWI diagnosis is given to those clients who consume excessive amounts of any/all fluids (e.g., water, coffee, urine, soft drinks etc.,) on a frequent basis, thus requiring fluid restrictions;

- The frequency of this level of impairment causes a disturbance in the client's ability to function in the social, emotional and biological domains of behavior.

Who is diagnosed with SIWI?

- The majority of clients diagnosed with SIWI are moderately to severely afflicted with psychogenic polydipsia and also have a diagnosis of schizophrenia (approximately 80% of clients diagnosed with psychogenic polydipsia have schizophrenia; approximately 1% of the general population have schizophrenia);

- The SIWI affliction can also be seen with people in the manic phase of bipolar disorder, intellectual deficits and severe personality disorder.

At What Point Would You Be Considered To Have SIWI?

- In simple terms, Self-Induced Water Intoxication (SIWI) is caused when a client drinks greater than 5% of his/her body weight within a 24-hour period on a regular, chronic basis (e.g., weekly basis). This causes an inability to function appropriately in the social, emotional and biological domains.

- A history of SIWI ranges from 4 months to 20 years onset and can also remain unnoticed. It is a "learned" addiction, the average period of time is a continuum of overdrinking behavior that is initially labeled as overdrinking abuse that subsequently increases to overdrinking dependence and finally ends with over- drinking addiction.

- Hyponatremia — the serum sodium level (Na) is less than 130 mmol/L. The normal range is 135-145 mmol/L. If a serum sodium level is less than 120mmol/L, this places the client at risk for seizures. Less than 106 mmol/L can cause coma and eventual death if left untreated.

Why do you drink too much?

The causes of overdrinking any/all fluids are unclear. Many factors influencing the development of psychogenic polydipsia and subsequent SIWI include the following:

1. The only correlation found why individuals overdrink any/all fluids is a family history

of alcoholism and/or the client has been a past/current habitual alcohol abuser (i.e., traded addiction);

2. A ritualistic way of coping with anxiety;

3. Overdrinking any/all fluids is due to boredom, weather related or obsessive-compulsive behavior;

4. A misconception and/or belief about water or fluids, in general a "more is better" attitude;

5. The client may be hearing voices telling them that it is good to overdrink and that it is healthy.

When Does a Client Commence Fluid Restrictions?

*   When the client overdrinks greater than 5% of body weight (e.g., 4 kg for males and 3.5 kg for females) in a 24-hour period.

How Does the Staff Manage/Treat SIWI?

*   Currently (i.e., 2003), there is no cure for severe psychogenic polydipsia and its habituated presentation of self-induced water (fluid) intoxication. For those clients with less severe forms of psychogenic polydipsia, the staff can attempt to control fluid intake. For those clients initially diagnosed with moderate to severe psychogenic polydipsia, a locked environment with staff control of client access to fluids is most often required;

    Staff monitor SIWI clients by weighing them 4 times per day (e.g., 7:30 a.m., 11 a.m., 3 p.m., and 7:30 p.m.);

*   The client's fluids are limited (e.g., no extra fluids provided during meals) if the client's weight increases (i.e., males greater than 4 kg and females greater than 3.5 kg). This is done to prevent the client going on fluid restrictions that entail being "grounded" on the water ward;

*   The consequences of going on fluid restriction depend on the weight gain. The client will be restricted to the water ward and his/her fluids will be restricted. This protocol is completed to give the client's body a rest.

When Does The Client Come Off Fluid Restrictions?

When a male client's weight is below 4 kg of the baseline weight. For example, for a baseline weight of 60 kg, the weight should be less than or equal to 64 kg. When a female resident's weight is below 3.5 kg of the baseline weight of 60 kg, the weight should be less than or equal to 63.5 kg.

SESSION I: PART 2
VISUAL DEMONSTRATION

- Recap Introductory Session 1

- Supplies needed: Scale, milk jug filled with water, cups

Procedure:

- Have three or four clients weigh themselves;

- After obtaining a base weight, have the clients hold a filled milk jug;

- Write on a white board the client's name and base weight then weigh the client while holding the milk jug.

When the above steps are completed:

- Have the clients pour out into cups the water contained in the milk jug;

- Have the group count the cups as they are being filled;

- Emphasize that this is the maximum amount of fluid they can consume. If they go over this amount, they will be placed on fluid restriction and restricted to the water ward;

- Ask the group, what is a healthy amount of water to drink per day? The answer is 8-12 cups over the duration of a day—NOT all at once;

- Separate 10 cups to show what is an acceptable amount of fluid intake per day.

SIWI SIGNS & SYMPTOMS

What Are The Signs & Symptoms of SIWI?

- The symptoms of SIWI are due to the imbalance of fluids in the body

- If sodium (Na) is below 120 mmol/L, marked symptoms develop which include: increased hallucinations/delusions

Question: *When you drink large amounts of fluids, do you feel any changes with your thinking or with your body?*

- Nausea, vomiting, headaches
- Dizziness, confusion
- Frequent urination, incontinence
- Slurred speech, blurred vision

Question: *Has anyone experienced any of these symptoms?*

- Feeling cold
- Decreased body temperature
- Edema
- Increased blood pressure
- Unsteady gait, seizures

Question: *Are you able to recognize when you are anxious?*

- Increased anxiety (general fears): Anxiety increases the likelihood that you will be less able to manage your fluid intake;
- Restlessness; unable to sit still, pacing, fidgeting, numerous posture changes;
- Sweaty; scared, agitated, decreased concentration, lack of interest.

Question: *What Can You Do When You Feel Anxious?*

- Go to a quiet area; learn assertive communication; talk to someone (express your feelings);
- Participate in activities such as structured games and exercise;
- Become involved in simple tasks, completing chores, going for a walk;
- Schedule your time with activities to keep busy in occupational therapy, physiotherapy, and recreation therapy;
- Ask for medication (PRN).

Question: *Do You Find Yourself Feeling More Irritable/Angry At Times?*

- More confrontations with co-residents; loss of control; yelling, swearing, threatening, name calling, throwing objects, hitting, short tempered.

Question: *What Can You Do When You Feel Angry?*

- Talk about your feelings with a staff member or someone you trust;

- Go to a quiet area of the water ward or community residence;

- Exercise: Use the exercise room in the recreation area—ask to go for a walk if you have ground's privileges;

- Participate in some activity that you enjoy—recreation therapy, occupational therapy, meditation, reading, watching T.V, playing pool;

- Challenge these aggressive thoughts with cognitive behavioral techniques (CBT—e.g., examining automatic thoughts); progressive deep muscle relaxation techniques; thought stopping, counting (1-8) visualizing the numbers to interfere with emotional arousal; diaphragmatic breathing exercises to control breathing rate;

- Ask for medication (PRN).

Question: *What Organs of Your Body Are Affected By SIWI? How Are These Organs Affected? (Use of Posters That Show the Organs Affected)*

- Kidney: unable to excrete extra fluids, infections, edema;

- Bladder: stretches and is unable to return to its original size, unable to fully empty as a result, urinary tract infections (UTI), incontinence, distended abdomen;

- Intestines: loose stool, increased number of bowel movements;

- Brain: severely increased fluid increases edema in the brain; decreased concentration and confusion; increased hallucinations/delusions; change in feelings (increased anxiety, irritability, anger); headaches; blurred vision; unsteady gait; seizures; coma, death;

- Heart: increased heart rate; increased blood pressure resulting in congestive heart failure (CHF).

Question: *How Does SIWI Affect Your Life Right Now?*

- Habitual overdrinking of fluids results in obsessive thinking about drinking all the time. Instead of participating in structured programs (e.g., O.T and RT outings) habitual over-drinking interferes with flexible thinking on a daily basis;

- Decreased ability for group involvement and social interactions—increased hallucinations/delusions; mood changes; decreased concentration; incontinence;

- Remain on locked water ward—less freedom; decreased amount of grounds privileges; premature aging of body organs, which is reflected in advanced aging appearance of the individuals diagnosed with psychogenic polydipsia; premature death.

Question: *How Would You Like Your Life To Change For The Better?*

- Move to an open unit; live in a community group home; have full grounds daily; be able to drink your favorite beverage in moderation when available instead of being on fluid restriction.

SESSION III
HEALTHY LIFESTYLE

◇◇

Purpose: To provide a nutrition education component to the SIWI Psycho-education Program.

Learner Outcomes: The clients diagnosed with psychogenic polydipsia will learn how much water our bodies need. In conjunction, the clients will learn healthy lifestyle strategies to control excessive water consumption.

Format and Content: Two 20-minute group discussion sessions. A visual presentation of common water and beverage containers as well as healthy food and fluid choices.

1. How much water do we need?
Healthy adults require at least (8 cups) of water each day to maintain good health. Individuals consume water in the form of liquids (i.e., juice, milk) and also in foods (i.e., primarily fruits and vegetables).

2. Why do we need water?
Body fluids are mostly water. These fluids flow through arteries, veins, and capillaries, carrying nutrients and waste products. Fluids fill cells and the spaces between them to keep healthy. Water is needed for many chemical reactions in the body. Water dissolves vitamins, minerals and other nutrients. Water helps to keep the joints lubricated. Water helps regulate body temperature and maintains the body's fluid balance. There is a delicate balance of minerals in our body. These minerals are called electrolytes, and they dissolve in water. Electrolytes include sodium, potassium and chloride. Electrolytes determine how much fluid stays in cells and how much remains outside cells. An imbalance is not healthy. Too much water inside cells is called edema or fluid retention. Excessive loss of water is called dehydration. The kidneys do most of the work of controlling fluid balance.

3. Is There Such a Thing as Drinking Too Much Water?
Yes, and it leads to a condition called "water intoxication" (i.e., self-induced water intoxication—SIWI). Water intoxication has been reported to range from a consumption of 4-10 L/day.

4. Symptoms of Water Intoxication
Nausea, vomiting, anorexia, dizziness, stupor, headache, blurred vision, incontinence, muscle cramps, tremors, convulsions, seizures, coma. Fluid ingestion in excess of the kidney's excretory capacity can lead to hyponatremia (low blood sodium levels). The brain dysfunction that occurs as a result of water intoxication can be due to hyponatremia, brain edema, intracellular potassium loss or all of these factors combined.

5. Visual Presentation During The Class
* Two water bottles of 1 L capacity each;
* One 8 oz. glass (250 ml);

- One 7 oz. Styrofoam cup (250 ml);
- One coffee mug (210 ml)
- One juice portion container (114 ml);
- One milk portion container (120 ml);
- One soda pop can (355 ml);
- One resource can (235 ml)

SESSION IV
STRATEGIES TO CONTROL EXCESSIVE WATER CONSUMP-
TION

1. Know what is the recommended daily fluid requirement for a healthy individual—8-12 cups of water per day (i.e., 1.5-2 L/day at least. Some clients may need more due to body size and physical activity).

    Note: Calculation used by Dietician: 30-35 ml of water per kg of body weight per day;

2. Know the good sources of water: juice, milk, Jell-O, broth, soup, fruits, and vegetables. Note: caffeine-containing beverages do not help in meeting water needs. Alcohol does not count toward meeting daily water goals;

3. Do not skip meals: Eat regular meals at a prearranged period of time each day;

4. Eat healthy snacks, if you must snack;

5. Keep busy: Get involved in regular, structured activities based in the hospital and community; more specifically, occupational therapy, recreation therapy, and vocational training. Daily exercise should become a routine; use the hospital recreation center and community recreation center (e.g., swimming, dancing). Outdoor exercise can include walking, jogging, running, roller blading, biking, skiing, and snow boarding; and

6. Eat fresh fruit and vegetables on a daily basis. The ingredients include: moderate water content, high fiber content, and high satiety value.

SESSION V
COPING STRATEGIES

1. What Can You Do To Alleviate the Urge To Drink?

- Structure your day with activities in vocational therapy, occupational therapy, recreation therapy, hobbies, and crafts;

- Learn a new hobby as both a short-term as well as long-term goal;

- Thought stop. Count (visualizing numbers 1-8) when you feel you must drink;

- Learn and complete twice-daily progressive deep muscle relaxation exercises. Beginning with 16 muscle groups, after extensive practice reduce (chunk) to seven muscle groups and finally chunk to four. Learn and complete on an as-needed basis diaphragmatic breathing exercises to reduce anxiety and increase attention, concentration, problem solving, and memory retrieval;

- Learn to divert obsessing about drinking. Instead, switch your thinking to other activities such as a beach scene, movies, skiing, swimming, running. Buy a rubber band, place it on your wrist, and snap the band to delay urges to seek out and overdrink fluids. Learn and practice cognitive behavioral strategies for psychosis (as 80% of patients diagnosed with psychogenic polydipsia are also diagnosed with schizophrenia);

- Some CBT techniques learned and practiced include restructuring, stress management via decatastrophization, and analysis of evidence; and

- Be able to routinely utilize these coping strategies to challenge the urge to seek out and overdrink any/all fluids.

2. What Kinds of Things Help You To Manage Your Water Drinking?

- The following information provides ways to decrease fluid intake: Drink in sips from a small cup; drink through a straw; chew gum; follow a prearranged routine regarding fluid ingestion; attend and comply with the behavioral management program and psychosocial rehabilitation semiweekly groups.

3. Which of These Techniques Have You Tried? Which Are Helpful? Why?

- Begin an unstructured, "open-ended" discussion from each group member about which techniques have worked for them;

- Why are these particular coping strategies successful for YOU?

4. Is Your Environment A Relaxed One? If It Is Not Relaxed, What Would Make It More Relaxing?

- Activities on ward or community residential living environments that are structured, fun and are both group and individual in format (e.g., drawing, reading, exercising, sending emails to friends, talking with other residents, friends and staff, playing pool);

- Activities off ward or community residential living environments that are less structured, such as: going to the mall, a movie, a club activity, and recreation center activities; and meeting friends and family members.

5. What Are Some of The Activities That You Do Throughout the Week (in and out of Living Accommodation)?

- Feedback is received from each client and a rationale provided why the client has chosen the specific activity(s).

6. What Kinds of Things Help You To Deal With Anxious Situations Now?

- Review the aforementioned coping strategies; Have a specified "down time" when anxious to commence the coping strategies to counteract anxiety.

7. Review Pertinent Topics to SIWI as Influenced by Questions from the Group Members

- Each of the five modules of the psycho-education training series is rotated on Tuesday and Thursday mornings. Additional topics of interest by the SIWI group can be incorporated into the psycho-education training format. In conjunction, other members of the multidisciplinary team can be utilized on an as needed basis regarding topics of interest requiring specific areas of expertise.

CHAPTER FIVE

RESIDENTIAL SETTINGS: A CONTINUUM OF CARE FOR CLIENTS DIAGNOSED WITH PSYCHOGENIC POLYDIPSIA

WHAT IS MEANT BY ORGANIZATIONAL DESIGN

Organizational design is decision making about the formal organizational arrangements, including the formal structures and the formal processes that make up an organization (Nadler & Tushman, 1988). According to the authors, the goal of the organization designer is to develop and implement a set of formal organizational

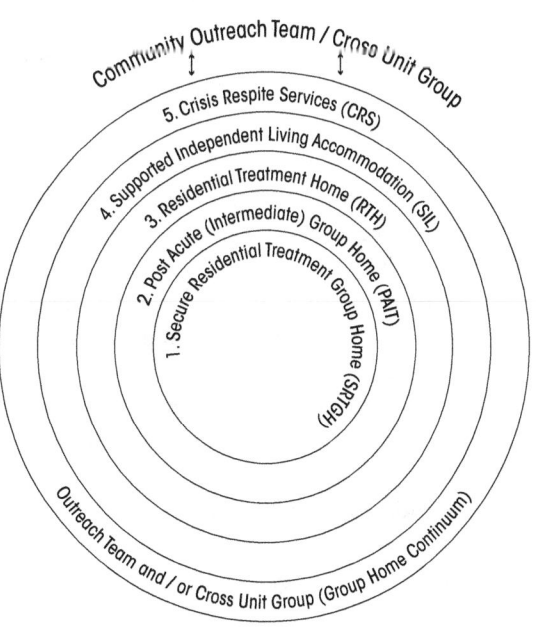

arrangements that will over time lead to a good fit among the different elements of strategy, task, individual, informal organization, and formal organizational arrangements. The authors further suggest that organizational design includes the following design elements:

1. Composition of organizational units;

2. Reporting relationships among units;

3. Other structural connections between units;

4. Organization-wide information, measurement, and control systems;

5. Organization-wide methods and procedures;

6. Organization-wide work techniques;

7. Subunit work resources (tools, materials);

8. Subunit reward systems;

9. Subunit physical work environment;

10. Individual job design.

Strategic grouping is the first and most important design step. Strategic grouping involves choosing the appropriate organization form at multiple levels and specifying the degree of specialization for each level. The degree of specialization is driven by information-processing requirements; the greater the task/environmental complexity, the greater the degree of required specialization. Strategic grouping decisions set the stage for *strategic linking*, a series of decisions focusing on coordination and control between interdependent pieces of the organization (Nadler et al. 1988).

Linking follows directly from grouping and, as with strategic grouping, must be accomplished at multiple levels of analysis. The issue is choosing the right set of linking mechanisms (e.g., outreach team) to deal with: (1) work flows between distinct units; (2) the need for disciplinary or staff-based professionals to have contact across the residential continuum housing the clients with psychogenic polydipsia, and (3) work flows being developed that deal with emergencies, crises, or other non-routine events. Accordingly, the conceptual thread across work flows, disciplinary linkages, and work flows under crisis conditions is work-related interdependence. In a group home continuum housing a clinical population with mild to severe symptoms of psychogenic polydipsia, the greater the task interdependence, the greater the need for coordination and joint problem solving. The more complex the degree of work/ task interdependence, the more complex the formal linkage devices must be to handle work-related uncertainty.

The simplest form of structural linking is the hierarchy: the formal distribution of power and authority. The hierarchy of authority follows directly from grouping decisions. Unfortunately, in the residential continuum treating clients with psychogenic polydipsia, the hierarchy is a limited linking mechanism. Because of an inherent cognitive/information-processing capacity, even modest amounts of task interdependence, exceptions, crises, or environmental uncertainty can overload the individual manager. This professional must deal with a multitude of problems over a 24-hour period, generated by this often chaotic clinical population.

When linking requirements begin to overload the first-level supervisor in the group home, other formal mechanisms must be used to complement the manager as a linking mechanism. These include *liaison roles* where more intense problem solving occurs between two liaison individuals who could be identified as point staff, either internally within the specific group home, or an external consultant, or an outreach team that floats among the various group homes of the continuum. These liaison roles serve as information conduits and initiators of overall problem-solving endeavors within the group home continuum. The liaison roles are also responsible for *enhanced information flows* (e.g., debriefing sessions, evaluating data collection, interfacing with novice staff; trouble shooting) and coordination among the group homes of the continuum. The liaison role is not usually a full-time responsibility but rather is done in conjunction with other activities.

Cross-unit groups include task-relevant representatives from the various group homes of the continuum who focus on particular clients and the specific presenting problems that are interfering with their progress through the treatment continuum. The cross- unit groups can be permanent, temporary, or ad hoc. Their objective is to assure that relevant expertise comes together to deal with their joint task or problem. In contrast to liaison roles, cross-unit groups provide a more extensive forum for information exchange, coordination, and the resolution of any conflict occurring between the respective group homes. At the outset of designing a group home treatment continuum for this clinical population, it is important to consider a cross-unit group as a representative subunit responsible for establishing and adjusting guidelines and processes that affect work flows across the group home continuum.

Lastly, when it is important to give equal attention to several critical contingencies (e.g., staff turnover) and when information-processing demands are substantial (e.g., evaluation of severe SIWI behavior), *matrix structures* are appropriate. On a positive note, a matrix structure improves coordination among multiple perspectives by balancing the power between dimensions of the organization and installing systems and roles to achieve multiple objectives at once. Matrix structures for the group home continuum treating psychogenic polydipsia have two chains of command. The first is the functional side, which is the day-to-day treatment programming that exists across the continuum. This requires scrutiny and continuous feedback looping regarding clinical decision making. The second is the administrative role, which coordinates the activities of the multidisciplinary groups across the group home continuum. It analyzes organizational problems from both a dynamic and an outcome focus. Information from both chains of command are processed from within and across functional treatment groups (e.g. job duties of multidisciplinary team) and coordination of organization-wide functions (e.g., organization dynamics and system evaluation).

The downside of matrix systems is their complexity. They require dual systems, roles, and controls, and the systems, structures, and processes must be developed to handle both dimensions of the matrix. The managers within this system must deal with the difficulties of sharing a common subordinate, while the common subordinate must interface with two bosses (Nadler et al. 1988).

DECENTRALIZATION

When designing a community group home continuum for this clinical population, the fundamental question in the decentralization-centralization debate is where decisions will be made in the organization. At what levels or at what locations within the organization will decisions occur? What will be the nature of the constraints or boundaries that are imposed on individual decision makers?

Decentralization has a number of distinct advantages. It promotes the processing of information among those organizational units, groups, or individuals who are closest to the work being performed. It also reduces the vertical information-processing requirements placed on the structure, since less information has to move up and down the hierarchy for decisions to be made. In practice, decentralization can promote responsiveness to local conditions, such as stabilizing a SIWI client recovering from a state of intoxication. In conjunction, decentralization provides the freedom that is needed to stimulate innovation, which, when dealing with chaotic behavior, requires flexibility to respond effectively to the intangibles that occur on a daily basis.

Conversely, there are clear disadvantages associated with decentralization (Nadler et al. 1988). Three major disadvantages are control, coordination, and cost.

Control involves the effective processing of information so that one level of an organization can ensure that another level is acting consistently with what is required. This involves the process of setting goals and standards, monitoring activity or behavior in comparison to those standards over time, and then taking corrective action (through feedback, incentives, or direct action) to ensure that the activity stays within acceptable limits of variation from the standard.

Coordination involves the processing of information so that various units operate to allow their activities to fit together to provide the required consistency of action across a set of organizational groupings. Coordination is usually necessary to achieve internal efficiencies or to provide consistency in relations with external consumers (e.g., family members).

Decentralization presents problems for both coordination and control. There is increased risk of loss of control or decrease in coordination to the extent that decisions are moved down in the organization, and only minimal boundaries are placed around the decision maker.

A third concern is cost, which involves both the direct cost associated with a design (e.g., salary, location expenses) as well as the indirect costs (e.g., management expense involved in maintaining minimal control over diverse activities). In conjunction, individual units may develop their own capacities that are duplicated in other group homes.

CENTRALIZATION

At the other end of the continuum is centralization. All decisions of any significance are made at one location in the organization, either by one individual, one group, or one organizational level. Any decisions that are made at the group home level are made only within very specific guidelines and according to standard operating procedures. Situations that must flow up the organizational hierarchy and don't fit the rules typically are treated as exceptions, which therefore must flow up the hierarchy to the point of central decision making.

The advantages of centralization are increased control and the potential to achieve enhanced coordination among units. There also may be direct cost advantages with making certain types of decisions at one point.

One disadvantage is that, if information is not at the central point, as is the case with a group home continuum, the resulting decision making may be slow, of poor quality, or highly unresponsive to the group home's immediate needs. In addition, centralization neither leaves room for nor encourages innovation, as much of the autonomy and potential to make decisions is taken out of the clinician's job function.

In regard to the centralization-decentralization continuum of organization administration, one must keep in mind the clinical ramifications of the client's quality of service provision. Recidivism can be used as an indicator of the quality of prior inpatient psychiatric services (HEDIS, 1993, as cited in Lyons, O'Mahoney, Miller, Neme, Kabat & Miller 1997). In this regard, Lyons et al. (1997) found that recidivism was related to the clients' severity of symptoms and levels of impairment in self-care. Frank & Brookmeyer (1995) examined "utilization review programs" and found recidivism was related to shorter stays and future recidivism. Gossett, Lewis, & Barnhart (1983) stated that the more chronic and severe the client's psychopathology, the more reduced the long-term adjustment and the higher the recidivism rate.

FACTORS REGARDING THE ADMINISTRATION OF A GROUP HOME PROGRAM FOR CLIENTS DIAGNOSED WITH PSYCHOGENIC POLYDIPSIA

Wolins (1974) suggested that a group home care milieu can be effective in creating positive change. His thoughts were expanded upon (Pazaratz, Randall, Spekkens, Lazor & Morton, 1999) to include:

1. Staff commitment—optimism about the possible outcome for the individual, no matter how deprived the background;

2. A sufficient length of stay to be meaningful to the person;

3. The opportunity to belong to an intimate unit of people, a place for family-like membership, in a way that does not compete with the natural family;

4. After-care support services;

5. Individualization of programs, especially in education. Clients are dual diagnosed (e.g., schizophrenia and psychogenic polydipsia) and many exhibit problems with attention, concentration, memory retrieval and problem solving;

6. The provision of adequate staff-client ratios for their safety and support;

7. The provision of backup resources for the client who becomes seriously suicidal, wildly aggressive or whose mental status requires a more secure setting for a period of time;

8. The opportunity to learn practical life skills that are transferable to each client upon discharge from the group home;

9. A definitive attempt to build group skills, strengths and cohesion by matching an individual with a group in terms of strengths as well as problem types (homogeneous living arrangement with other residents diagnosed with psychogenic polydipsia); and

10. Staff members on the multidisciplinary team who bring to the task a special kind of tolerance. The staff working with SIWI clients should be chosen for their sense of personal security, demonstrated competence with this demanding clientele, and interest in carrying through with life-skill teaching activities regardless of the hardships brought on by the clinical population.

PREVENTING INSTITUTIONALIZATION IN THE COMMUNITY

In this section, institutionalization can be viewed regardless of whether it houses a clinical population in a traditional institution or a community setting. Two ways to focus on institutional environments entail the structural features and the functional features (Landesman, 1988). The *structural features* of a residential facility refer to such characteristics as location, size, ownership (i.e., public, proprietary, or nonprofit) and staff-to-client ratio. *Functional features*, in contrast, indicate the actual way a residence operates. Examples include the amount and quality of interaction between staff and clients, the types of activities in which clients engage, and the degree to which an individual's personal needs are met. Two group homes housing clients diagnosed with psychogenic polydipsia may be similar in terms of their structural features, but they may differ substantially in how they function. They may have the same number of clients and staff members. In the first home, the staff-to-client ratio may be perceived as inadequate, due to the severity of the clients' water addiction and the frequency of isolating the clients in seclusion due to the intense supervision required by one or two clients. In contrast, in the second group home, because it has less severely addicted clients and less interventions caused by SIWI, the staff members are better able to provide the special needs to the overall group home client population. Even though the structural features of size and staff-to-client ratio of these two homes are equivalent, the functional consequences for the clients are quite different. There are four negative functional features that make residential settings institutional in nature. They are rigid administrative organization, behavior of direct care staff toward residents, resource utilization, and relationships with others outside the residence (Landesman, 1988).

Rigid Administrative Organization
Generally the administrative structure in traditional institutions is cumbersome and complicated. There is usually a hierarchical reporting structure, with primary decisions about residential care made at the top and carried out at the bottom. Direct care staff who perform their jobs well are usually promoted into positions that take them away from working with clients, at which they have excelled. This dynamic maintains a system in which the least experienced and least ambitious staff have much of the front-line responsibility for the residents' quality of life.

A first-rate care provider may not necessarily be good at supervising others, managing programs, or fitting into a larger bureaucracy. Traditional institutions typically have many rules and detailed procedures. Despite the many hours that are spent writing and rewriting procedures, most staff members openly admit that many of these procedures and operating policies are not followed. There is often a "them against us" mentality in large institutions, a well-defined division of staff into direct-care workers versus supervisors, professionals, and administrators. This has often manifested into a ripple-down effect providing a rationale for programs being offered that are less effective than they should be.

Clinicians complain that the direct care workers do not consistently carry out programs to achieve specified objectives. The direct care workers complain that many clinicians and administrators hold expectations that cannot reasonably be met within the existing setting. In many instances this is true, as the behavioral programs for the SIWI clients can often be too time consuming, too technical, or too tedious for direct care staff to conduct. Alternatively, professional teams select behavioral goals that appear insensitive, superficial, or excessively ambitious to the direct care staff (e.g., the SIWI client will reduce fluid restrictions by 80% in six weeks).

The administrative organization of most institutions is one in which change occurs very slowly because each proposed change must be submitted for careful review within the hierarchical system before translating it into action at the level of the residential unit. By having decisions made at a distance, those responsible for enacting these decisions naturally feel uninformed and remote, and are relatively unmotivated to comply enthusiastically. Consequently, the administrative and organizational features that contribute to institutionalization include depersonalization in decision making, rigidity in organizational policies, and lack of autonomy among direct care staff. All of these factors have obvious implications for the administrative environment of community residential programs.

Behavior of Direct Care Staff Toward Clients Diagnosed with Psychogenic Polydipsia
The primary fault in the behavior of direct care is lack of sufficient social interaction with clients. Findings from Landesman's (1988) observational studies indicated that the amount of time direct care staff spend in social interaction with clients (which includes all forms of social exchange) averages 10%-15% of their total time on the job! The majority of direct care staff believe that this low amount of interaction is the result of the staff shortage in institutions. According to Landesman (1988) there is contrary evidence: merely adding more direct care staff will not significantly improve the situation, and she cites numerous authors to defend her position (Baumeister & Zaharia, 1987; Knight, Weitzer, & Zimring, 1978; Landesman-Dwer, 1981; Landesman-Dwyer, 1984b). She further states this purported lack of direct care staff should be called the *myth of understaffing.* Moores & Grant (1977) describe this as the *avoidance syndrome.* In their opinion, being highly sociable with clients and attending to their social needs are not staff behaviors that have been highly valued or emphasized in traditional institutions. Looking at this identified problem more closely, very few procedures deal directly with how much positive social interaction should occur between staff and residents. Landesman (1988) further states that another misconception is limited social interaction being caused by the unresponsive client, the *myth of the unresponsive client.* The premise suggests that when staff members do not detect a social response from clients, they gradually stop paying attention to the clients.

There are several characteristics about social interactions in institutions. First, they tend to be very brief and infrequent, and second, they often seem impersonal and "pat." Demonstrations of patience, concern, genuine interest or pleasure by the staff can often be muted. Third, almost all direct care staff show evidence of being good natural teachers. This ability, according to Landesman (1988), is seldom employed. Regardless of how distant or abrupt a staff member may seem during routine activities, there are moments when that same individual displays his or her ability to teach, to encourage, or to provide constructive feedback to the clients. The situations in which this natural teaching seems to occur are those that are unplanned or spontaneous and are not associated with any formally assigned staff teaching activities. Landesman-Dwyer & Berkson (1984) state that what is clearly missing in institutional environments is true appreciation of the significance of informal talking, everyday teaching, the sharing of feelings, or just having fun together.

Insufficient Resource Utilization
The concept of resource utilization extends beyond the issues of where services are delivered and who controls them. Resource utilization may also include making the most of the human talent available within a residential facility. Institutions function primarily by compartmentalized daily activities into many distinct areas. This requires assignment of responsibility to many different staff members. Employees hired to fill a specific job are rarely able to participate in activities not included in their job description. Landesman (1988) has stated that if the natural interests and abilities of direct care staff were utilized more fully and in a flexible fashion, then the opportunities for staff to become more personally involved and more enthusiastic in initiating positive changes should increase. The idea that the individual personalities of the direct care staff could, and should, contribute to creating a dynamic, unique "home environment" is

foreign to most institutional settings. The reality is that most staff members are viewed as inter-changeable. This is supported by the practice of reassigning staff from their regular living unit to other units at the last minute, with little or no orientation to the new environment, whenever absences or vacancies occur. Similarly, staff often leave their home unit and go to a new one to obtain a better work schedule or to be promoted. The functional consequences of treating staff in this depersonalized way can be problematic and needs to be remedied.

Lastly, Landesman (1988) has stated that, to utilize resources effectively, community residences first need to consider what types of social and physical assistance could be beneficial. Next, the availability of resources within the group home and surrounding community should be ap-praised, recognizing the possibility that there may be some areas in the community that enrich the lives of the clients, staff, and family members. She further states that clear responsibility for resource management is important to establish and to keep current. It is meaningful to re-member that variety and novelty are desirable elements in a community residence, and that the interests and needs of residents should influence the acquisition and use of resources.

Limited Relationships with Others
Treatment facilities in community residences often criticize institutions for their rigidity in deal-ing cooperatively with other service agencies. This is a two-way complaint! Staff in institutions claim that community-based professionals and service providers are not sufficiently responsive, knowledgeable, or cooperative with the institution. Accordingly, with emotions often running high, such interactions bias the outcome, and in turn reinforce the initial prejudices of each side and prevent forming closer ties. As Landesman (1988) states, to prevent segregation from occurring, community residences can establish a broad network of relationships with individu-als and community agencies. These contacts should be open, frequent, and mutually beneficial. If administrators insist on knowing about all contacts that staff members and residents have with others, then such social links to the community are likely to be limited or guarded.

WHY QUALITY OF CARE DECLINES IN THE COMMUNITY

Why do some of the best community residences eventually become more institutional in char-acter? There are usually three issues involved: (1) they are not prepared for the difficulties as-sociated with the long-term operation of a residential program; (2) they have no built-in means of self-evaluation; and (3) they lose some of their own sense of internal direction and personal goals, accepting instead the standards and programs of other agencies or advocacy groups (Landesman, 1988).

Difficulties in Long-Term Operation of a Facility
Community residences experience the daily problems and frustrations inherent in any group living arrangement, often exacerbated by the shifting needs of individual residents and new de-mands generated by the clients, their families, and/or case managers. Landesman (1988) states that a number of contributing factors include staff migrating to other jobs, returning to school to advance their education, and facing limitations in salary and opportunities for promotion.

Program expansion may decline in quality after their administrators and advisory boards decide to expand service provision. After succeeding with one residence, these individuals are often encouraged to open a second, then a third, or more new residences. The managerial skills needed to succeed in operating community residences in a cost-effective and organizationally sensible manner may be quite different from those skills that contributed to success in the first model program. More specifically:

- When leaders shift their attention away from the first community residence and the clients there—directing their energy into opening new facilities, getting to know new clients, training new staff, and finding ways to make things run more efficiently and with less effort—the first residence may suffer from neglect;

- The subsequent community residences in expansion efforts often seem to be carbon copies structurally, but functionally they may lack the spontaneous, creative, high levels of activity and caring energy that characterized the first community residence;

- The leaders often show little or no awareness of the decline in the day-to-day quality of life. Since these individuals are very busy with expanding their programs, they are at risk for losing touch with daily activities and the subtle aspects of social life that are vital for real success; and

- Once success has been achieved in the planning and early operation period of the new homes, the administrators want to move on, not realizing that equal creativity in problem solving and especially in problem avoiding is vitally needed to maintain a home environment that promotes continuous, but not stagnant, high quality of care for those who live and work there.

Inadequate Self-Evaluation

Landesman (1988) states that because community residences exert much effort in proving to outsiders that they can provide high quality services, they are less motivated to be highly introspective. Self-critique is often feared as a negative process that may demoralize staff, families, or clients. This may also reflect the doubts that many staff experience daily about their competence to handle many of the complex, sensitive, and important matters that are central to their jobs. Because cooperation is vital to success in residential settings, self-evaluation may be a constructive way to prevent programs from becoming stagnant or merely reactive to outside criticism.

Loss of Self-Direction

Landesman (1988) states that a third quality decline in residential programs is the loss of self-direction. This may be caused by the need to comply with standards established by others. Such external directedness may lead to less active engagement of staff, families, and community. Variety and trial and error are needed when they occur in a caring and committed environment. Excessive structural regulations constrain creative new program efforts and eventually contribute to a situation in which blame for substandard care can be placed outside the facility. This is comparable to the negative situation in institutions in which individuals, including staff, administrators, and clients, lose their motivation to try to improve things. Landesman (1988) states external standards should become increasingly based on the functional aspects of what occurs and how residential programs actually support the development and well-being of clients, rather than the current reliance on structural components. Landesman states the problems with primary reliance on structural features are: (1) adherence to these may be used to substitute for (that is, merely comply with stated standards) more individualized adjustment of a group home to the varying preferences and needs of those who live there; (2) the minimal costs of meeting these may be so high that homes have virtually no extra funds to initiate programs of their own; and (3) their own goals for program development and resident progress are subordinated to external standards.

STRATEGIES FOR PREVENTING INSTITUTIONALIZATION

There are three ways to help prevent suboptimal or declining care, each of which can be implemented within the present system and with existing resources (Landesman, 1988). The first is to encourage service providers and recipients to evaluate things on their own. When the incentives for self- appraisal come from within a group home, the process is likely to be more effective. The multidisciplinary staff in a group home designed for co-occurrent disordered clients should be able to shape the evaluation process and make changes on an ongoing basis (i.e., formative evaluation). Ultimately it is they who are the ones to decide on and implement changes.

The second way to prevent suboptimal or declining care entails providing a functional objective for every structural regulation. For example, if the staff-client ratio is mandated (a structural regulation), then the corresponding functional consequences should be stated. Perhaps the functional intent is that each client receive a certain amount of individual attention from staff on a daily or weekly basis, or that there be sufficient coverage to handle emergencies. Once the functional objectives become as clear as the structural objectives, then a substitute or an equivalency formula could be used for group homes with exceptional circumstances (e.g., severe SIWI clients). This would not mean an exemption from compliance with a policy, but instead offering to group homes flexibility in how to chose to meet an objective. Many homes would continue to adopt the general structural recommendations because these appear reasonable and helpful. Others may prefer more freedom in developing their own proposals. In such a system, all group homes remain accountable for their own outcomes. This would mean that compliance with a conventional structural recommendation would not be sufficient evidence that the objective was achieved.

The third way to prevent suboptimal or declining care would entail the promotion of more interaction among staff in community residences. Staff treating the SIWI client in community residences need to be in contact with other programs treating psychogenic polydipsia, which are also striving to provide a high quality program for persons with this clinical problem. By frequent sharing of ideas as well as complaints, the multidisciplinary team members treating this clinical population are likely to feel supported and to develop professionally. If staff members have the opportunity to visit other residences, they are more likely to observe both positive and negative features they can translate into action in their own programs. In sum, institutionalization refers to sub-optimal, routine, and depersonalized care that can occur anywhere. Serious efforts must be made to prevent institutionalization from affecting the community residential treatment milieu. This may be achieved by frequent self-evaluation, improvement of existing formal regulations and evaluation activities, and expanded efforts to create a peer network for direct care providers.

TREATMENT PLANS FOR CLIENTS DIAGNOSED WITH PSYCHOGENIC POLYDIPSIA

Treatment plans in community rehabilitation settings designed for clients with psychogenic polydipsia have generally been constructed to expose the individual to transdisciplinary assessments (e.g., psychology, occupational therapy, physiotherapy, vocational therapy, recreation therapy, medicine) and for the results of these assessments to be integrated into an overall treatment plan. Historically, day treatment programs for this unique clinical population housed in community group homes have been fully capable of providing the services of the aforementioned disciplines. Consequently, when developing and staffing a day program, an assumption can be made that the necessary disciplines are represented in the treatment team. It is further assumed that the provision of a multidisciplinary team will allow the respective clients adequate access to clinical services and personnel to increase the respective potential for a positive outcome.

An alternative approach to the development of the treatment plan is as follows: Instead of staffing a day treatment program by disciplinary means, the programs first consider a formal assessment of the likely needs of its clientele in functional terms then provide treatment staff who can accurately address those needs. This distinction is conceptually and in practical terms more client centered. The obvious criteria for this clinical population would reflect the client's severity index (i.e., mild, moderate, severe) of the psychogenic polydipsia diagnosis. The real needs of the clients may have been held in abeyance and in deference to a traditional view of rehabilitation as discipline centered (versus client centered). Recreation therapy, psychosocial rehabilitation, and life planning are three examples of ancillary treatment approaches that are sorely needed in the treatment of psychogenic polydipsia.

It is the author's contention that day treatment programs for this clinical population be staffed and managed with a direct appreciation for the identified functional needs, along with an investigation of these needs for each client they are to serve. The day program thus becomes a comprehensive problem-solving treatment model, staffed by individuals familiar with the clinical needs of the client population. In this regard, a treatment plan is really a descriptive problem list, the "problems" (e.g., overdrinking any/all fluids) being those day-to- day barriers that the client with psychogenic polydipsia must overcome to make a meaningful advancement toward greater independence and discharge to a less restrictive community residential setting. The treating clinicians in the day program will have training specific to a given discipline. However, the decision to treat should not be solely bound by administration of treatment that is proper for that discipline. More specifically, the therapists should self-critique their repertoire of skills and determine whether those skills and teaching abilities coincide with the respective client's needs. Post-acute rehabilitation has been moving in this problem-solving direction for the past 20 years, although several philosophical barriers, with regard to which discipline performs a therapeutic activity, have remained in many treatment milieus (e.g., occupational therapy taking over group counseling that has been traditionally the responsibility of social work and psychology).

In summary, it is the author's opinion that treatment plans should not necessarily be structured according to various traditional disciplines. Rather, a day program must first assess the additional needs of each SIWI client (e.g., vocational training, speech-language pathology, advocacy for government subsidies, legal counseling) and personnel retained who can meet these needs. Proper resource management should clearly prevail when a prioritized treatment plan is established for this clinical population. In addition, regarding the triad treatment rehabilitation model discussed in earlier chapters (e.g., medication, behavioral management, psychosocial), the additional needs manifested by each respective client that cause significant impact on the client's eventual ability to progress to a less restrictive living accommodation must demand sufficient attention and effort by the multidisciplinary team in each residential milieu. Clients' access to the day program is finite and boundary specific. Their time on program must be used in accordance with the barriers or problems that have the greatest negative impact on their recovery (e.g., over drinking any/all fluids). For example, this may cause, at some level of the treatment modality, the living skills training being deferred, as it is perceived to be of lower priority than having the client gain control over patterns of habitual overdrinking. Nevertheless, it is the author's belief that prioritization should be actively attended to and monitored closely in the day program to avoid a treatment bias that neglects other important considerations in the client's recovery.

Clinical Case Management A poorly designed treatment intervention can lead a client diagnosed with psychogenic polydipsia down the "rehab road to failure." Similar failure can occur when the client's care is not properly managed. In cases of severe self-induced water intoxication, this may precipitate the possibility of several rehabilitation professionals assuming accountability for solving the problem. This begs the questions—Who is in charge of the treatment plan? Who determines the prioritization of problems to be addressed? Who assists the client in the treatment decisions and the effect (i.e., the use of limited resources)? To provide some clarification, Hembree (1985) defined the clinical case manager's role:

The combination of activities designed to insure appropriate use of medical care facilities, improve quality of care, control or reduce costs, insure proper referrals, provide primary care, and manage patients' episodes of care, disability, and rehabilitation" (p.11)

In a day treatment setting, the multidisciplinary team involved in the treatment effort for each client diagnosed with psychogenic polydipsia requires a single point of accountability to exist regarding the overall direction and ultimate outcome of a client's treatment program. Case management services are facility based for this particular clinical population. That is, case management functions in the day rehabilitation program as the service accountable for out-come (Evans & Preston, 1990). It is prudent to have a case manager assigned to each client in a day program setting, as the possibility exists that nonprogram personnel (e.g., private physicians, family members) may exert significant influence on the overall rehabilitation process and inadvertently function as the case manager.

In summary, clients with psychogenic polydipsia living in a community residence require case management services for their respective day programs. Case management significantly reduces the risk for errors of omission in treatment planning, reduces cost overruns, and greatly improves the likelihood for appropriate use of and access to resources (Dixon, Goll, & Stanton 1988).

A Group Home Continuum to Treat Psychogenic Polydipsia During the past two decades, commencing in the early 1990's, community-based group homes have gained wide acceptance as a resource for the care and treatment of clients diagnosed with psychogenic polydipsia. Residential group homes located in the community are facilities where a number of residents live under the supervision of staff members. These homes are distinguished from other residential care facilities by (a) small size—no more than eight occupants; (b) relative to more traditional hospital institutions, there are few restraints on the movement of clients and on their interaction with the surrounding community; and (c) reliance, to a certain degree, on community resources (e.g., recreation facilities) to provide adjunct services to meet the overall needs of the client diagnosed with psychogenic polydipsia.

The institutional model does not fit this particular type of group home. The staff are seldom in a position to exert 24-hour "close supervision" over the activities of the clients diagnosed with psychogenic polydipsia. Typically, the clients are functioning in the mild-moderate/severe range of psychogenic polydipsia. More specifically, their fluid-seeking behavior entails a need to overdrink any/all fluids. They have usually been transferred to the group home as either a step down from a more restrictive (higher staff-client ratio) environment, whether it be a formal institutional setting in a hospital or health care facility or from another more structured group home facility, where observation of overdrinking any/all fluids was made by staff somewhat familiar with the specific presenting features of psychogenic polydipsia. That being said, community group homes geared to treating psychogenic polydipsia have to adopt distinctive approaches oriented to their special circumstances (i.e., monitoring excessive fluid seeking and ingestion). In the absence of intensive supervision and a controlled physical environment, as is the case in less restrictive group home environments, the staff must rely on indirect, nonauthoritarian ways of influencing residents, which can be a challenging and at times stressful job with this demanding clinical population.

A description of the physical environment is in order, prior to describing each group home on the continuum of care. The writer gratefully acknowledges Shostack's (1987) comments about the makeup and physical layout of group homes.

A group home's physical surroundings affect the feelings of the clients about themselves, the staff, and the living milieu of the group home itself. They expand or curtail opportunities for recreation, study, and cooperative relationships. Minor inconveniences such as inadequate closet space and a cramped dining room can create human-relations problems that increase the risk of increased fluid consumption with this clinical population.

Good ventilation and comfortable temperatures in the group home are important for the health and disposition of the clients. Air conditioning has major advantages; it reduces irritability and emotional overarousal and facilitates sound sleep. At the very least, the group home should invest in high quality fans to help the clients and staff through the summer heat. Needless to say, accident hazards should be eliminated. Loose steps, poorly lit stairwells, sharp edges on kitchen equipment, and exposed wires are things to assess and remedy.

Kitchens in group homes require oversized stoves, sinks, and refrigerators. Adequate storage and work space is essential. A good idea is to purchase two refrigerators, one for general food storage that is off limits to the clients and a smaller one that clients can utilize as in a normal family setting.

The dining area should be roomy and used as a gathering place for group discussions and visits with friends and family members. There will be times when clients prefer quiet time to read, watch television, or talk with friends. The common rooms of a group home are heavily used for recreation, organized group activities, or just hanging out. It is recommended that two common rooms be provided. One should be available for noisy and social activities such as listening to music, playing pool, and watching television. This room should be furnished inexpensively and informally. The second common room is a quiet room for passive activities. These might include reading, chatting, and playing board games.

Appropriate sleeping areas contribute to the therapeutic milieu. Bedrooms serve as a private retreat from the tensions of group life. Bedrooms should be well ventilated, lighted, and cool in hot weather. Rooms that are cramped evoke tension among the occupants, as are rooms that are unequal in size. In this regard, staff should be alert to potential problems. Long-term clients may haze new clients and make requests for changes in room assignments as a test to the group home authority structure and/or to maintain a feeling of ownership regarding the physical living area. In either case it is in the staff's best interests to maintain the harmony of group home.

An adequate number of bathrooms reduces conflict in a group home. This is particularly true in the mornings and evenings when the clients are beginning and ending their day. Efficient use of bathrooms includes utilizing other space for personal care activities. Extra mirrors and vanity tables enable female clients to dry and set their hair elsewhere in the house.

When furnishing a group home for this specific clientele, the "institutional look" should be avoided. Beds should not be of the institutional type; closets and wooden wardrobes for storing clothes are preferred over more institutional metal lockers. Bedrooms should differ somewhat; however, overall size should be approximately the same to avoid unnecessary conflict. Clients should be allowed to individualize their rooms, such as bringing their own possessions to be placed around the room.

Furnishings should be as attractive as possible so that clients can identify proudly with the home, develop an appreciation for the surroundings, and feel good about inviting friends and relatives to visit. Dressers and/or foot lockers are needed for adequate storage space. There should be sufficient desks and lamps to encourage reading and comfort level. In selecting furniture, the effect on the clients must be kept in mind. More specifically, the dining room table should be large enough to avoid crowding that evokes negative interaction among the clients. The availability of two or more dining tables permits seating choices for the clients and helps to avoid bickering. There should be enough chairs and tables in the common rooms to avoid territorial arguments.

Desks in the bedrooms facilitate a work area for each client and allow a more formal area for working correspondence. A bookcase encourages the clients to read and have an area for placing material that might be otherwise left on the floor.

The availability of a backyard for leisure activities encourages clients to spend free time around the group home, where they can be observed and supervised, if need be, by the staff. It offers an alternative to congregating on the front steps, which can be irritating for a passer-by. The outdoor area can be equipped with sturdy benches and tables for picnics, games, and passive relaxation. If the backyard is not very large, it is useful to surround it with a hedge to protect the privacy of the neighbors and the clients of the group home.

A birdhouse or a bird feeder is an inexpensive way of stimulating interest. A staff member or volunteer may even enlist the help of a client in some gardening that is required around the group home.

Quarters for the Group Home Staff

Residential group homes in the community are staffed 24 hours per day. It is imperative that the staff have a comfortable working area removed from the common area of the group home to allow them to complete their reports and other necessary paperwork with privacy. Those staff covering the "graveyard" shift (e.g., 11 p.m.-7 a.m.) must have adequate quarters from which to work and are necessary if the staff are to perform their therapeutic roles effectively.

Working with clients diagnosed with psychogenic polydipsia can be a tension-filled role over a prolonged period of time. The clients have a tendency to relapse and remit in their fluid drinking habits, which causes boundaries to be tested incessantly (e.g., group home rules), especially when the client has sodium depletion and is SIWI (i.e., hyponatremia). As a consequence, the group home staff working on a shift basis with this difficult and often perplexing clinical population require working quarters that are comfortable. The environment must allow them amenities such as a refrigerator, a television, and a separate room for office space for those persons who relieve them. Requirements for office space vary depending on the staffing pattern of each group home and whether the group home's supervisor and social worker have offices at some outside location.

If they are located at the group home, they require, as a minimum, a room for writing counseling correspondence, filing records, and conferring with staff members. Other professionals affiliated with the group home (i.e., psychologists, occupational therapists, psychiatrists, recreation therapists, vocational workers, and family physicians) may have to work in a common area, albeit in a private domain pertaining to their respective discipline's requirements, for such duties as individual and group counseling, confidential phone calls, and meeting with other professionals and family members.

Lastly, which staff members and how many are needed to run a successful group home are the final questions to be answered before describing each group home's working paradigm. Despite the small size and apparent uniformity of the group homes, there can be striking differences in their staffing patterns. Staff roles are combined in many ways, and a staffing pattern that works in one group home may be unsuccessful in another.

There are some traditional tasks that are essential in a residential group home located in the community. The group home's treatment paradigm for the clients diagnosed with psychogenic polydipsia must be developed and directed by a competent staff member familiar with the unique presenting problems of this clinical population. There must be a least one person qualified to evaluate the treatment needs of each client, arrange necessary treatment services, serve as liaison with agencies outside the group home continuum, counsel clients and family, and manage each client's unique case requirements. Trained professionals in a variety of disciplines pertaining to rehabilitation of this clinical population are essential to supervise residents on an everyday basis. Several staff members must take on educational, recreation, housekeeping, maintenance, clerical and other support tasks of the group home.

GROUP HOME/TREATMENT CONTINUUM

1. Secure Residential Treatment Group Home (SRTGH)

2. Post-Acute Intermediate Treatment Group Home (PAITGH)

3. Residential Treatment Home (RTH)

4. Supported Independent Living (SIL)

5. Crisis Respite Group Home

6. Outreach Team

Comment: Strategic Links and Liaison Roles promote interdependency between group homes and effective evaluation.

Staff members

Director of the Group Home Service Continuum

The author is indebted to A. Shostack's insightful comments in his text, "Group Homes for Teenagers: A Practical Guide" (1987). The director of the group home service continuum designs each group home's treatment approach to be based on the diagnostic level (i.e., mild, moderate, severe) of the clients with psychogenic polydipsia. This professional selects and trains the staff members and decides which clients are admitted for care. This person, along with the group home supervisor, represents the group home in relation to the placement of the client from another group home within the continuum mentioned above or an external referral source (e.g., hospital, health care clinic). The director's position should be full time and located outside the working parameters of interacting intensively with the clients on a daily basis. If this is not followed closely, there can be a tendency for the director to lose objectivity and the long-range view of the overall program needs of the group home continuum. If the director's relations are too close with the clients, the director's ability to function in the role of an objective, treatment-oriented professional may be negatively influenced. That being said, a director who works out of a distant office surrenders a measure of knowledge and control. In this regard, this professional should feel comfortable delegating more authority to the respective group home supervisors of the continuum. Some directors feel that distance sustains their objectivity, reduces burnout, and lends them an aura of authority that helps to maintain discipline in the facilities.

Program design issues for the group home continuum have a myriad of challenges for the director to consider. More specifically, how will the clients with psychogenic polydipsia be evaluated and selected? What services will be provided across the continuum of service, how often, when, where, and by which disciplines? What will be the duties of each staff member? How and to what degree will the clients' lives be structured? What will be the group home's policy of clients' social conduct, family visits, room assignments, telephone use, finances, chores, and incentives?

An overall treatment plan for each residential facility, including admission and discharge criteria, should be prepared and juxtaposed with the other group home treatment plans of the continuum. This will facilitate each group home conducting its respective program in a systematic manner and reduce knee-jerk reactions in response to crises and unanticipated requirements. Generally, a written treatment design for each group home helps to maintain a continuity of services when staff members are replaced and serves as a basis for staff training and periodic evaluation of the program. The recruitment and training of staff and the collection of information about salaries and fringe benefits paid to comparable workers in other facilities are duties of the director. It is helpful to prepare a brochure describing the group home's objectives, facility, and service provision *in toto* and in regard to the group home continuum. The brochure should be distributed to placement agencies within the catchment area of the group home continuum, prospective clients and their families, community organizations, family physicians, and local government officials.

A handbook for clients provides a framework of shared information and expectations for staff and clients. A handbook should inform the client about such issues as legal status, the role of the group home continuum in successfully treating psychogenic polydipsia, staffing responsibilities, and services and policies of the group home. Useful items to include are (Shostack, 1987, p. 53): a welcome to new clients; the history of affiliations and objectives of the group home; the address and phone number of the facility; the name, address, and phone number of the placement agency and a brief statement of its responsibilities and procedures; the names, titles, and duties of the staff; a description of the group home's treatment and support services, recreation and educational-vocational opportunities, and family services; rules such as sharing of chores, visiting privileges, and use of telephone; and the locations of community facilities that clients will be using, such as the local community recreation center, library, bus terminal, and shopping areas. It is not recommended that the handbook be burdened with long lists of rules, penalties, and rewards. This information could precipitate feelings of anxiety and cause a relapse of overdrinking fluids. In conjunction, the group home's behavior management program details are left to be distributed in a separate document at a time when the client can be more formally approached by the staff and the behavior management program explained in a reassuring manner.

Responsibilities after the Group Home Is Operational
Once the group home is fully operational, the director's principal task is to develop a therapeutic social milieu. Formalization of rules pales in comparison with the successful supervision of staff/clients, which is an art as well as a set of technical skills. Day-to-day life in a residential group home must be influenced with flexibility and subtlety. The director, in close alliance with the group home supervisor, has to keep in touch with the feelings and opinions of the staff, clients, outside contact agencies, and the parents of the clients. The director's functions in a fully operational group home include the following (Shostack, 1987):

Relations With the Group Home Supervisor
The director must maintain a supportive working relationship with the group home supervisor and, to a more limited degree, with the multidisciplinary team. The director should meet with the group home supervisor at regular, prearranged intervals and submit monthly and annual reports. The preparation of an annual budget by the director for the facility also gives the group home supervisor an opportunity to evaluate program needs and plans. The director, in consultation with the group home supervisor, prepares annual budgets and represents the group home in negotiating the periodic review of its licensure. This also includes preparing for periodic agency evaluations, submitting required documentation/reports pertaining to the operational standards of the group home, and meeting with licensing officials and other representatives of official importance to the operation of the group home.

Administrative Responsibilities
The administrative responsibilities for the group home continuum are usually shared with a bookkeeper, an administrative assistant, a chief of maintenance, and other pertinent managers of resources to successfully run a group home enterprise. These responsibilities are likely to be overseen at each respective group home by the group home supervisor.

Continuous Refinement of the Group Home's Policies
The director and group home supervisor should revise the group home's policies continuously

in the light of experience and changing needs. Policies must be adapted as the group home's clientele change, old rules become outdated, and new standards are imposed by external sources.

Supervision of Staff

The director recruits and has trained paid staff and volunteers regarding the treatment protocol of each group home in the continuum. The "counseling" of staff members is a distinct feature of the director's role. This job function is a prime requirement due to the nature and degree of emotionally labile behavior by a client who is water intoxicated! The clients' day-to-day functioning—the incessant testing of rules/boundaries of the respective group home environments during and after the "honeymoon period"—can cause tensions for staff and clients alike. The crucial importance of self-awareness, emotional stability, and objectivity in dealing with this clinical population cannot be overstated! In this regard, the group home supervisor can often be too close to the problem, requiring a more objective, arm's length approach from the director.

Selecting Clients for the Group Home Treatment Services

The director reviews the files of potential clients prior to meeting with the group home supervisors to discuss whether the referral meets the admission criteria for the group home continuum. If so, an interview is set up with representatives from the referral source, the client, and any family members. A preplacement visit with the client and his family and a consult meeting are arranged with the prospective group home staff to debrief them on the candidate for admission.

Treatment Services

The director, in consultation with the respective group home supervisors, selects, monitors, and evaluates the performance of the ancillary professional staff hired to "flesh out" the treatment needs of each client admitted to the group home continuum. These professionals can include psychiatrists, family physicians, dentists, recreation and occupational therapists, physiotherapists, neuro-psychologists, speech-language pathologists, and vocational rehabilitation workers.

Relations with Community Agencies

The director nurtures good relations with neighbors of the group home, civic groups, the news media, police, recreation facilities, and other community elements. The director may also accept speaking engagements, attend community functions, prepare press releases, organize public relations activities, and represent the facility in associations.

Termination of a Client

The decision to terminate a client prior to completing a course of treatment is made by the director in conjunction with the group home supervisor.

Miscellaneous Tasks The director exerts a subjective influence by being easy to talk to, glad to lend a hand, fair, trustworthy, and a role model for staff and clients. He or she uses authority with judgment and restraint to minimize the grievances and insecurity that fester in group home settings. The director, as well, has to demonstrate strength to challenge when necessary, to maintain discipline, to correct staff members, even when such actions evoke anger and complaints.

Group Home Supervisor
The duties assigned to the group home supervisor for this community-based facility usually entail (Shostack, 1987):

* Helping the director design services and everyday routines for the group home;

* Training and advising the various staff and ancillary professionals brought in on a case-by-case basis regarding the treatment of psychogenic polydipsia;

* Counseling staff members to help them cope with personal and work tensions;

* Evaluating potential clients regarding the entrance criteria of the group home;

* Developing and updating treatment plans;

* Advising professionals who conduct individual and group counseling;

* Liaison with all aspects of client movement within the group home continuum;

* Arranging hospital admissions for clients who relapse and require intensive medical and/or psychiatric treatment;

* Advising the director concerning the need for a client's termination in the program or transfer to another group home within the continuum of services; and

* Planning aftercare services for clients who are being discharged from the residential program.

Psychologists and Psychiatrists
Psychiatrists and psychologists are necessities in the treatment of psychogenic polydipsia. The medical and behavioral management/psychosocial rehabilitation needs of this clinical population are best served by these two disciplines in an overseer/advisory function. The severity of the psychological disturbances and the ebb and flow of the treatment progress of the clients are factors considered in planning psychological services. Typical duties of psychiatrists and psychologists include advising on the content of the group home's treatment program, evaluation of potential and current clients, advising on individual treatment plans, individual and group counseling, treatment of client's medication regime, training staff members, and counseling them concerning work-related and personal problems. The group home continuum should hire both disciplines on a contract basis to provide a predetermined set of skills pertaining to the treatment requirements of the respective clients.

Nursing Staff

It is necessary to have nursing staff available, if possible, hired as permanent part-time employees, to work onsite at the various group home facilities of the continuum. It is important that the nurse on shift understands each client's medication protocol and is apprised of the client's behavior during the previous 24-hour period. The nursing staff can also coordinate the completion of the client's periodic evaluation of psychogenic polydipsia via the Virginia Polydipsia Scale and the St. Louis Modified Water Intoxication Scale. They also oversee the medication compliance issues and liaison responsibilities with the psychiatrist and family physicians.

Paraprofessionals

Paraprofessionals (e.g., diploma graduates in rehabilitation from a community college) who do not have licensure requirements to practice their discipline exert a deep influence on the clients they treat on a 24-hour daily basis. The continuous and close contact with the clients exerts a very deep influence on the overall treatment milieu. The manner in which these staff members implement policies and treatment plans vitally affects the outcome of the respective programs of the clients. The paraprofessional working with clients diagnosed with psychogenic polydipsia is often confronted with the acting-out behavior of an intoxicated client while receiving little immediate support from the professional staff. As a result, the job requires resourcefulness, self-confidence, and strength of character. The contagious effect of a water-intoxicated client on peers living in the group home can create aggressive and confrontational behavior. Paraprofessionals are often thrust into a mediation role during their shift, which includes preventing aggressive behavior from escalating and preventing theft, bullying, extortion, sexual harassment, and hazing.

Their responsibilities also include fire prevention, the exclusion of unauthorized persons from the premises, monitoring the behavior of visitors, and guarding against the introduction of illegal drugs, alcohol, and any other fluid of substance (e.g., water jugs). Depending on the staffing requirements of the group home in the continuum, the paraprofessional roles combine mentoring, informal counseling, and teaching rudimentary things such as personal care and housekeeping chores. The paraprofessionals also help with the cooking, chauffeuring, and maintenance of the building. Lastly, the paraprofessionals are responsible for observing the behavior of clients (e.g., weighing protocol), reporting each client's progress, and bringing the clients' needs to the attention of the professional staff.

Support Staff

Support positions for the group home continuum include cook/housekeepers, clerical workers, and maintenance personnel.

Cooks/housekeepers

These workers are employed in either a full-time or part-time capacity. The role of the cook/housekeeper allows the paraprofessionals more time to interact with clients and to recuperate from their emotionally demanding duties. A skilled cook can improve the quality and variety of food served in the group home and can reduce food costs by preparing meals from primary ingredients rather than serving more expensive canned products.

Clerical Workers

Clerical assistance (office administrator) should be utilized when possible in all of the group homes of the continuum. Specific job responsibilities include phone duties, typing duties, duplicating (photocopying), facsimile work, filing, and taking minutes at meetings. If the budget does not permit full- time clerks in each group home, dividing a full-time equivalent position into two equal part-time jobs should enable each group home to have regular access with a clerical support worker. Lastly, clerical chores for direct care staff consume time that could be spent on substantive work with the clientele, necessitating the clerical position to be made a budget priority.

Maintenance Worker

Group homes are buildings that are usually older (i.e., 30+ years) and thus require continual patching and replacement of worn-out equipment. Living quarters and furnishings receive rough use that requires frequent painting, repair of laundry equipment, unclogging of drains, and re-gluing of tables and chairs. Such work is aggravating, expensive, and time consuming. The group home continuum should make a maintenance worker position a budget priority, as outside craftsmen come at high cost to make major repairs.

Ancillary Professionals Occupational Therapist/Recreation Therapist/Physiotherapist/Vocational Worker

Individual treatment plans (ITP's) that are developed for clients of the group home continuum should include a brief description of each client's psychological, medical, vocational, and general symptomatic behavior pertaining to the DSM-IV primary AXIS I-V diagnosis. In conjunction, long-term treatment goals outside of the medical, behavioral management, and psychosocial rehabilitation paradigm will most often entail interfacing with one or more of the aforementioned professionals (e.g., occupational therapy, recreation therapy, physiotherapy, vocational rehabilitation). As well, short-term objectives, covering periods up to three months, often require treatment intervention from one or more of these professionals. These disciplines are vital in providing well-rounded and meaningful treatment programs and should be under contract and available across the group home continuum.

Staff Relations

The author gratefully acknowledges the following information as suggested by Shostack (1987, p. 78):

• Staff conferences, conducted at least once per week, are a must for all group homes of the continuum. The director and group home supervisor should make time for frequent informal exchanges with the paraprofessional staff;

• Periodic written evaluations (e.g., semiannual) of all employees contribute to honesty in staff relations and help bring problems into the open where they can be analyzed objectively;

- As members of the treatment team, the paraprofessionals should be consulted in planning the group home's policies, admitting and terminating residents, developing ITP's, and evaluating the progress of the clients;

- Group home supervisors should review periodically the authority and responsibilities assigned to staff members to ensure that they are clearly delineated and understood by all parties;

- The group home supervisor, director, and social worker should spend a proportionate amount of shift time in the group home, including some evening and weekend hours;

- Interpersonal conflicts should be the subject of staff supervision sessions; and

- Group home supervisors should express support for staff members. A word of praise, a commendation witnessed by the clients, and a luncheon invitation build trust, respect, and loyalty among the staff.

Group Home Continuum

Strategic Links

A series of decisions focusing on coordination and control among interdependent work activities of the group home continuum;

Linking is accomplished at multiple levels of analysis: work flows between distinct units; the need for disciplinary or staff-based professionals to have contact across the residential continuum; and work flows being developed that deal with emergencies, crises, or other non-routine events.

Liaison Roles

- When linking requirements begin to overload the first level supervisor in the group home, other formal mechanisms must be used to complement the supervisor as a linking mechanism;

- Liaison roles are established where more intense problem solving occurs between two liaison individuals who could be identified as point staff. These individuals are identified internally within the specific group home; an external consultant, or an outreach team that "floats" among the various group homes of the continuum; and

- The liaison roles serve as information conduits and initiators of overall problem solving endeavors within the group home continuum;

- The liaison roles are responsible for enhanced information flows (e.g., debriefing sessions, evaluating data collection, interfacing with novice staff, troubleshooting, and coordination among the group homes).

Cross-Unit Groups

- Cross-unit groups include task-relevant representatives from the various group homes of the continuum who focus on particular clients and their specific presenting problems that are interfering with the individual's progress through the treatment continuum;

- The cross-unit groups can be permanent, temporary or ad hoc;

- The objective is to assure the relevant expertise comes together to deal with their joint task or problem. Cross-unit groups provide a more extensive forum for information exchange, coordination, and the resolution of any conflict occurring between the respective group homes; and

- A cross-unit group is a representative subunit responsible for establishing and adjusting guidelines and processes that affect work flows across the group home continuum.

1. Secure Residential Treatment Group Home (SRTGH)

Facility
This is a first stage step-down group home for clients diagnosed with moderate-moderate/severe levels of psychogenic polydipsia, ostensibly those individuals discharged from an institutional environment (i.e., hospital setting) or a community based facility that accommodates hard-to-manage clientele. The license capacity for this group home in the continuum is no more than eight residents. The need for a seclusion room in this facility is a reflection of the client's continued relapsing-remitting cycle. This cycle is frequently problematic (i.e., SIWI) but still reduced from institutional frequency, thus allowing discharge to a less institutional, albeit locked, community facility.

Staffing Model
The director of the group home continuum oversees staffing configurations with input from the group home supervisors. The multidisciplinary team should entail: group home supervisor, full time; family physician, psychiatrist, and psychologist, on contract; nursing, permanent part time; paraprofessionals, support staff, and clerical, full time; ancillary workers, on contract; and other professionals (e.g., pharmacist, lawyer, dentist) on an as-needed basis.

Admission Criteria
A full review of each client's file from the referring agency or institution should be appraised by the director and group home supervisors prior to a preliminary conference with the candidate, his family or trustee, and referral agency representatives. A thorough examination of the severity of the candidate's psychogenic polydipsia and other mental health concerns should be discussed. It is recommended that the level of psychogenic polydipsia severity is quantifiably appraised. The use of a standardized assessment instrument (e.g., Virginia Polydipsia Scale; St. Louis Modified Water Intoxication Scale) to provide data as an adjunct to the subjective commentary by the referral agency representatives is recommended at this

point in the referral process.

If there is no such information available, the referral is placed on hold until the candidate can be assessed. This is also the case with a full psychiatric history or mental status examination and any other medical or psychological testing that is deemed appropriate to assess the individual. It is imperative that the group home staff receive any/all written documentation regarding the potential candidate's current and historical mental and physical functioning. All information provides clues to help treatment success!

If the candidate is turned down due to a lack of clinical documentation or does not meet the criteria of this particular group home of the continuum, another meeting will be held with the director and group home supervisors in attendance. The information imparted at the initial preadmission meeting will be debriefed and recommendations made regarding how, when, and where the candidate could be better placed. The information is provided to the referral agency to allow any loose ends to be resolved, and another meeting may be scheduled with the referral agency.

When the candidate is accepted for admission, it is understood that a long-term relapse (e.g., 2-4 weeks) could precipitate a referral to an inpatient emergency hospital bed outside of the group home continuum. The client's return to the group home is dependent on the information provided by the hospital, and the final decision to readmit the client is made by the director of the residential continuum.

Each client in the group home continuum receives an ITP that is developed and updated on an ongoing basis, throughout the treatment duration at the particular group home facility.

At the secure residential treatment group home, the emphasis is on developing tailor-made treatment programs involving medication to stabilize the client's mood, a behavior management program to reduce the client's propensity to seek out and overdrink any/all fluids, and a psychosocial closed group program of which attendance is mandatory and one-to-one counseling (e.g., CBT techniques taught) is practiced. In conjunction, any other treatment resources vis-à-vis the ancillary professionals (e.g., recreation therapy, occupational therapy, vocational rehabilitation services) are included on an as-needed basis, in addition to other professional resources required to rectify a client's particular dilemma (e.g., legal matter).

Data are collected and collated on an ongoing basis, and staff decisions about client access to fluids is influenced by the person's level of addiction at this point in the treatment program. Base weighing procedures and frequency of fluid restrictions are the cornerstone criteria from which clinical decisions are made. In conjunction, ongoing quantitative data collection via standardized assessments (e.g., Virginia Polydipsia Scale) provides objective information about each client's progress. A thorough review of the charted notation concerning the individual is completed by the client's identified case manager (i.e., paraprofessional) and the group home supervisor. This information is collated and condensed and brought to the weekly staff meetings to provide additional information from a subjective standpoint of the multidisciplinary team. This is very valuable information to keep track of and allows themes of drinking patterns to be identified as well as emotional "buttons" (i.e., discriminative stimuli) that provoke the client and precipitate fluid seeking and overdrinking behavior.

The multidisciplinary team meets formally on a weekly basis regarding each client on program. In conjunction, "hand-over" times throughout the 24-hour work schedule provide an opportunity for informal information to be passed along and decisions made about the client's requests for increased freedom.

The SRTGH group home is a first stage, step-down facility, just below institutional staffing levels and as a result continues to use some of the institutional rules to allow generalization to occur regarding client confinement. More specifically:

- **Level 1:** Client is confined to the group home;

- **Level 2:** Client is allowed to leave the group home with staff supervision but must stay on the property;

- **Level 3:** Client is allowed to leave the group home property but is still under supervision by a staff member; and

- **Level 4:** Client may leave the group home property without supervision but only for a predetermined period of time.

Weighing each client four times per day is mandatory. A base weight should be administered upon arising (e.g., 7:30 a.m.) and after the client voids. This is followed by additional weighing at 11 a.m., 3 p.m., and 10 p.m. or thereabouts. Subsequent decisions about client confinement are based directly on the person's ability to control his or her fluid intake.

Each day the client is involved in structured ongoing activities, with each activity lasting 15-30 minutes, at which time a break is provided and the individual is allowed to stay and continue or seek out alternative activities of the client's own choosing. Clients should be provided four or five structured activities throughout the day. They are required to sign in and out of the activity and encouraged to keep a file (notebook) on each activity.

As treatment progresses, the desired outcome is achieving reduced frequency of self-induced water intoxication and consequent fluid restrictions, as well as reduced group home confinement due to aberrant behavior. Data collection should indicate, over a treatment period of less than three years, a slow, steady progression of increasing control by the client over the need to seek out and overdrink any/all fluids.

Discharge Criteria
This first stage step-down residence from a more formal institutional psychiatric environment (i.e., closed, locked hospital unit) is not to be relegated to a custodial or warehouse role, but

rather a dynamic treatment atmosphere, where gains are expected to be slow but steady. The tedium of the clients' relapsing-remitting treatment response can be very frustrating for the staff and clients alike, causing friction and disappointment. However, understanding the nature and course of this illness at the outset can help to reduce burnout by the staff.

Steady, albeit slow improvement in reducing the client's frequency of SIWI is one indicator of treatment success and should be reinforced continuously via verbal praise, token reinforcement, and group support during the psychosocial interventions. Other indicators include increases in self-esteem, personal care, attention, concentration, memory and problem-solving abilities. Staff consensus on client improvements and a greater willingness to allow the individual off-site activities that are not as closely monitored as previously is another example. Lastly, the quantitative data from the daily reports, weekly meetings, and test results from the standardized assessment instruments provide a triangulated information flow from different sources and approaches to treatment outcome.

Liaison from the Outreach Team Toward the end of the treatment duration at the secure residential treatment facility (SRTGH), the outreach team is introduced to the client and the client's support system. During this transition period, discharge to a reduced level of care is discussed, and/or return to an institutional facility if the client has not shown improved ability to control overdrinking any/all fluids. It is expected that a client diagnosed with moderate to moderate-severe psychogenic polydipsia should, with time, improve and reduce the need to overdrink. At this time the outreach team, in conjunction with the SRTGH group home supervisor and with sanction from the director, develops a discharge strategy.

More specifically, if the client is to be transferred to the post-acute intermediate treatment group home (PAIT), a two-week transitional admission will be negotiated as the bed capacity warrants. Timelines will be set up for a transitioning period of the current treatment program to allow generalization to the PAIT group home treatment protocol.

After the two-week visit leave, a formal meeting will be held with the SRTGH and PAIT group home staff representatives, the client, and the client's support system (i.e., family/guardian). At this time the outreach team will preside and offer support and/or a referral to the cross-unit group if the need arises (i.e., family problems with referral, specific areas of concern with the client vis-à-vis the placement and other residents). The outreach team allows the transitioning and blending from the SRTGH to the PAIT group home by helping to resolve any internal problems perceived as being roadblocks to the transfer.

Once the client has been successfully discharged from the SRTGH to the PAIT residence, the client's treatment plan is transferred, and any internal problems with living adjustment becomes the responsibility of the PAIT facility. A three-month window is kept available for return to the SRTGH residence pending availability of a bed. Typically, the client's failure at the PAIT residence will be the intransigence of the excessive fluid drinking (i.e., SIWI) and extensive relapse time, making discharge to a more secure setting the only clinical option.

2. Post Acute (Intermediate) Treatment Group Home (PAIT)

Facility
This group home has a slight reduction in the staffing-resident ratio. It remains a licensed eight-bed, locked facility with a seclusion room for those clients who relapse and have SIWI problems. There is one major difference with its intermediate care provision. This facility is more accommodating for discharge to or from higher and lower-staffed care facilities, referring clients diagnosed with psychogenic polydipsia. More specifically, the occasional client will be discharged prematurely from the SRTGH facility or its equivalent and relapse, thus necessitating a transfer back to the original referral source. Conversely, a client may be transferred directly to the PAIT group home after the preadmission conference and adjust quickly to the treatment program, thus necessitating a re-evaluation of treatment needs and imminent discharge to a reduced level of care.

Staffing Model
The staffing model is ostensibly the same as the SRTGH group home, with one difference. Due to the greater flexibility built into its referral system, the PAIT group home will make use of the outreach team's liaison role to a much greater degree than the SRTGH group home. As a consequence, referral to the cross-unit group for more in-depth intervention is warranted more frequently. Such a referral would be warranted if, for instance, a client has been transferred from a group home within the continuum and problems have developed regarding a transfer back to the client's original group home or to another group home in the continuum, whose staff are uneasy with the transfer (e.g., client mix does not match well). The cross-unit group would be utilized if these scenarios' problems were not easily rectified and required extended mediation from this specialized unit.

In conjunction, greater flexibility of client referral will require a staffing complement that is comfortable with higher client mobility and less stability in day-to-day operations. Such flexibility is not everyone's cup of tea, especially with this clinical population. It is a wise group home supervisor who carefully selects the staff after providing a thorough orientation of this group home's mandate. If major problems occur, it is also wise to request the services of the cross-unit group, sooner rather than later, as the gains made with the specific client might be lost in episodic relapse due to an ongoing problem within or between group homes.

Admission Criteria A candidate for the PAIT group home has most often a moderate level of psychogenic polydipsia. This includes a relapsing-remitting cycle that is longer in the remitting cycle than exhibited by a client in the more severe range. In conjunction, the candidate has received a thorough assessment from the referral agency, which, by the data available, indicates a movement in treatment progress. The more thoroughly the candidate's current level of functioning is reviewed at the preadmission conference, the less chance exists of an inappropriate referral. This is a significant point, as a candidate should be at the contemplative stage of understanding the nature of his or her illness. The subsequent treatment program (i.e., ITP) during the first three months will further reinforce the client's comprehension of the cause-effect nature of the relapsing-remitting cycle. This understanding should allow a steeper learning curve to occur over the duration the client requires this level of staff involvement.

Treatment Program The group home continuum follows the biopsychosocial model discussed in earlier chapters, utilizing a combination of medication, behavioral management, and psychosocial rehabilitation techniques to facilitate change in thinking and adaptive behavior.

At PAIT each client is provided a case manager (i.e., paraprofessional) who oversees and monitors the ITP of the client. Formal weekly staff meetings with the client in attendance examine the strengths and needs of the respective programs and their challenges (e.g., conflict between clients, abusive behavior to staff by resident and family, resident's aberrant behavior in the community).

The cross-unit group, group home supervisor, and director of the group home continuum can be expected to be utilized to a great degree if an inappropriately placed client is having difficulty adjusting to this particular group home and/or transfer problems have developed for whatever reason. Treatment progress is monitored both subjectively and objectively, once again triangulating all assessment information, to obtain the best possible answer to the myriad of questions posed by each client's maintenance of his or her overdrinking any/all fluids.

Treatment can generally last from 12 months to three years. The client's clinical progress is measured in frequency of SIWI, fluid restrictions, and stabilization of other psychiatric symptoms. Generally the consequences for infractions include reduced privileges inside and outside the group home.

Discharge Criteria One obvious indicator of readiness for discharge is the client's frequency of SIWI and fluid restrictions, which have become markedly reduced as a result of the positive influence of the treatment programming. At this point in the treatment progress, the client is considered functioning at a mild level of psychogenic polydipsia. The relapsing-remitting cycle is much reduced, with the remitting portion being much longer in duration. The client comprehends the cyclic nature of psychogenic polydipsia and has developed a cadre of appropriate coping strategies that have been assimilated throughout the course of treatment.

In concert with the client's observable changes regarding less frequent symptomotology and greater control of the psychogenic polydipsia, the multidisciplinary team has a consensus, or near-consensus opinion, that the client is ready for discharge to a less restrictive living environment. This goes hand in hand with a reduced staffing complement and more freedom for the client to come and go from a group home with fewer barriers and a more normalized lifestyle. Collation and examination of the client's subjective and objective data from the PAIT group home usually confirms the staff consensus regarding readiness of client discharge.

A discharge meeting is called that includes the client, the client's case manager, multidisciplinary team members, client's family or guardian, the group home supervisor, the liaison team, and representatives of the receiving group home in the continuum or external group home.

The treatment program is discussed and a four-week trial placement arranged. At this time the client's treatment regimen is taught to the group home staff to allow generalization of skill development, easy transition to the new facility's treatment protocol, and adjustment to the other clients.

Liaison from the Outreach Team

If the client has difficulty during the trial placement period, the outreach team is utilized to resolve problems. The receiving group home may request an extension of the placement period or after the four weeks decide the candidate is not acceptable. This information is imparted at a formal preplacement meeting verbally and in writing with rationale and with input from the liaison team. In this instance the representatives of the outreach team present their findings and a decision is made. If the candidate is not accepted for placement, he or she is returned to the PAIT group home for further treatment. If the outreach team's recommendation supports the group home's request for an extension of the preplacement trial period, contingency arrangements are made by both the PAIT and the receiving group home.

If any problems exist beyond the competence of the outreach team, the cross-unit group is contacted to conduct further examination of the problems and, if need be, the director of the group home continuum is involved. Lastly, when the discharge is approved and the client moves to the new location, follow-up is provided by the outreach team to facilitate any transition problems that might occur.

3. Residential Treatment Home (RTH)

Facility

An RTH group home is developed for clients assessed with marked symptoms of psychogenic polydipsia—chronic water seeking behavior and/or diagnosed with mild psychogenic polydipsia. Clients must be able to harmonize well with the surrounding neighborhood with a minimum of visibility and traffic. An upper limit of six beds is recommended, keeping in mind that one or two beds will occasionally be vacant. The group home will be an open environment without restrictions to access of any/all fluids. As mentioned earlier in the chapter, good ventilation and comfortable temperatures are important for the health and disposition of the clients. There is no designated seclusion area, and any acting-out behavior will be handled *in situ* by the staff on duty.

An inability to curtail an escalation of client aggression will result in the crisis respite resources (CRR) team being contacted, which could lead to transfer and seclusion in the PAIT or SRT-GH group home. For further detailed information on the physical layout of the RTH group home, please review the earlier pages of this chapter.

Admission Criteria

The admission criteria for this particular group home requires objective and subjective analyses of the candidate's current psychiatric and functional status. This entails psychological testing, including a quantitative assessment of the candidate's current level of psychogenic polydipsia (i.e., Virginia Polydipsia Scale) and an examination of subjective charted notes of any past or current information on the candidate's level of psychogenic polydipsia.

Ideally, an acceptable candidate does not compulsively overdrink any/all fluids or, alternatively, has been treated for an extended period of time in the more restricted group homes, (e.g., SRT-GH; PAIT) and has successfully reduced the tendency to overdrink any/all fluids and is currently at a mild level of psychogenic polydipsia. The candidate is deemed capable of being redirected by the staff and therefore presents a much reduced risk factor for relapse. The remission-relapse cycle is very broad, with the former being extended in time (e.g., 6-12 months) if not longer. Secondly, as done in the previous living accomodation, a functional assessment is completed by the occupational therapist, including activities for daily living (ADL), personal time management, community resources, schedules and calendars, giving and receiving directions, banking, computer use, and a host of other skills.

The data are collected, collated and presented at a preadmission meeting with attendance by the candidate, his family or designate, the group home supervisor, professional staff debriefing the assessments, paraprofessional staff, and representatives from the referring facility. A decision is made to accept or reject the candidate. If the person is accepted, a four-week trial period is begun, at the end of which another formal meeting is held to debrief the committee about the candidate's behavior during the trial period and decide on formal admission. If the candidate is rejected, a rationale is provided with recommendations quantifying, in logical order, what change has to be done, in what period of time, to increase eligibility.

Staffing Model

The staffing complement should include the following disciplines: group home supervisor, paraprofessional staff, contracted ancillary staff as required, nursing (permanent part time), professional staff contracted as required, and support staff.

Group Home Supervisor The group home supervisor should be a full-time position with the incumbent having the necessary competence in administration ability, clinical knowledge pertaining to rehabilitation, and, more specifically, the treatment of psychogenic polydipsia. The treatment program for the RTH group home should be developed keeping in mind the array of services in the continuum (i.e., SRTGH; PAIT) and the other designated facilities treating this clinical population, but operating externally to the group home continuum (e.g., open and closed hospital wards; community clinics).

The group home supervisor, in conjunction with the director of the residential services and the other group home supervisors of the continuum, will design an RTH treatment program with the following issues addressed:

• Hiring competent staff from various multidisciplinary professions and paraprofessions (i.e., licensing not required to practice) who will be taught treatment techniques germane to this unique clinical population;

- The reduced level of psychogenic polydipsia will place additional complexities on service provision when intangibles crop up. This is in part because of the greater independence of the clients at this facility and their dual diagnosis (e.g., schizophrenia and psychogenic polydipsia);

- How the candidates will be evaluated and selected, and the basis on which their respective circumstances are prioritized;

- What services will be provided, by whom, how often, when, and where;

- The duties of each staff member and whether cross-training will be allowed outside of the discipline's focus;

- How the day-to-day life of the client will be structured; and

- The RTH group home's policy on curfews, family visits, room assignments, telephone use, chores, incentives, etc.

The treatment program should be prepared in writing prior to the first client being admitted. This allows a systematic process to be followed and early problems resolved quickly before they become unmanageable.

The group home supervisor will be in continuous contact with the other group home supervisors of the continuum, both formally and informally, to ensure transitioning problems are reduced. The RTH group home houses high functioning clients who are at an advanced stage of being treated for psychogenic polydipsia. Keeping in mind this is a traded addiction at its extreme and is a co-occurrent disorder (e.g., schizophrenia and psychogenic polydipsia), special attention should be made regarding any behavior that appears to indicate a relapse is occurring or about to occur. As mentioned in the other group home facilities, once the RTH group home is in full operation, the group home supervisor's primary task is to develop a therapeutic milieu. Life in this particular group home, due to the high functioning level of the clientele, requires influential leadership, flexibility, and empathic gestures to staff, other officials external to the group home continuum, clients, and their parents.

The group home supervisor should meet with the director of residential services at least weekly at the beginning of the treatment program and, later on, no less than monthly. In conjunction, the RTH group home supervisor should meet with the other group home supervisors on a weekly basis to share information and review file information on potential candidates. Lastly, the preparation of an annual budget for the facility also gives the group home supervisor an opportunity to evaluate program needs and plans.

Paraprofessional Staff
The paraprofessional staff are typically a qualified rehabilitation worker or social services

graduate from a two-year community college diploma program. They can also be part-time baccalaureate students in aligned professional programs such as psychology, social work, psychiatric nursing, occupational therapy, and recreation therapy.

They are hired to do shift work and are trained by the group home supervisor and ancillary professional disciplines regarding the treatment protocol of this dual diagnosed clinical population.

Staffing is required seven days per week. Shift hours are generally 7 a.m.-3 p.m., 3 p.m.-11 p.m., and 11 p.m.-7 p.m., with some overlap of shifts to provide time for the exchange of information and staff meetings. A competent paraprofessional shift worker can, with time, become very adept at completing routine shift functions specific to this clinical population (e.g., daily weigh-ins, completing routine assessments pertaining to the level of psychogenic polydipsia, interaction with family members and professionals assigned to complete contracted duties, and arranging for appointments as necessary).

Clearly, on-the-job training is essential for paraprofessional workers. In addition to learning about the symptom sequelae of clients diagnosed with psychogenic polydipsia, they must learn and be familiar with the group home's policies and routines. They should receive training in leading group discussions, providing informal counseling, recognizing the symptoms of psychiatric illness and psychogenic polydipsia, and managing peer group relations.

It is strongly recommended that a new staff member develop a "buddy system" with another more experienced staff member and spend at least the first four weeks observing and assisting the experienced worker before assuming personal case work responsibilities. Simultaneously, during this learning period, a professional staff member (e.g., group home supervisor) should provide systematic instruction covering all aspects of the new employee's job that do not lend themselves to on-the-job training. In conjunction, to encourage a seamless transition from another job and clinical population by the new employee, there should be structured in-service training for paraprofessional shift workers, which includes regular staff discussions, formal lectures by the psychologist on psychogenic polydipsia and DSM IV-AXIS I & II behavior, and arrangements to participate in workshops offered by outside agencies.

Ancillary and Professional Staff
Psychiatry, psychology, social work, occupational therapy, recreation therapy, family physician (G.P.), vocational rehabilitation worker, clergy, part-time nurse, and others may be hired on a contract basis as needed.

Their duties vis-à-vis the respective clients obviously depend on the nature of the therapeutic need and the contractual arrangement. This formal arrangement is usually established after a request is received by the group home supervisor by way of the group home's weekly team meeting. Hiring a part-time nurse to oversee medication and act as a conduit with the physicians, other professionals, and representatives of community health care facilities (e.g., admission/discharge duties) can help the internal treatment dialogue run smoothly and efficiently.

Three essential treatment components of the RTH group home include education, recreation, and health services. Not only do these services benefit directly the health and development of the respective clientele, but, by influencing clients' self-concepts, relationships, and attitudes, they affect the outcome of all other program activities. For example, if the need to seek out and overdrink any/all fluids is not resolved, this will aggravate psychological distress and impair the individual's relations with other clients. From the writer's perspective, when the RTH group home is being developed, it is imperative that budgetary allotments for professional and ancillary staff are provided and placed in an operational funding category that cannot be appropriated for other uses!

Support Staff
Support positions at the RTH group home include housekeeper, clerical worker, and a maintenance position (part-time). Such workers free up time for the clinical team from routine tasks, allowing the team to concentrate on shift duties and other essential resident-specific responsibilities. The housekeeper, apart from completing household chores, can double as a cook, at least on a part-time basis. A housekeeper in the cook role can improve the quality and variety of food served in the group home and teach cooking skills to those clients interested in furthering their understanding of preparing meals from primary ingredients. The clerical worker provides support for the group home supervisor and the staff complement by performing typing duties, filing, faxing, emailing/photocopying documents, and providing a conduit between the workers and clients (e.g., family communications).

The maintenance worker is hired on a part-time basis to keep the group home upgraded regarding living quarters, painting, repair of laundry equipment, unclogging drains, re-gluing tables and chairs, etc. The maintenance worker, depending on the number of facilities involved, can be shared throughout the group home continuum on a fairly equitable basis. Keep in mind upgrading work can be aggravating, expensive if done by someone unfamiliar with home repairs, and time consuming. This particular staff role is important and should not be forgotten in the budget.

Treatment Program
The treatment program of the RTH group home follows the biopsychosocial model of intervention. Each client is evaluated for psychogenic polydipsia and general mental status, and a personalized treatment plan is developed by the multidisciplinary team.

The paraprofessional shift worker takes on the role of case manager for a specific client and provides feedback on a weekly basis at the team meetings, debriefing any/all strengths and needs manifested by the resident during the treatment protocol.

The case manager oversees the development of a client's behavioral management program, involvement in semiweekly psychosocial group meetings, formal one-to-one counseling sessions, and informal daily interactions.. Medical intervention is also carefully monitored by this individual with the support of the part-time nurse. Charting, data collection, formalized assessment and evaluation, and subsequent changes in the treatment program are also supervised by the case manager, with sanction from the multidisciplinary team and support from the group home supervisor.

Perceived problem resolution as endorsed by the multidisciplinary team (i.e., reduced tendency to overdrink any/all fluids) requires careful discharge plans to orchestrate an appropriate transition to a less structured staffing model. Or, if the client regresses (e.g., family crisis) a transfer to a more secure residential setting, ideally within the group home continuum.

Discharge Criteria to Supported Independent Living – SIL
A client seeking discharge to a reduced level of care such as supported independent living (SIL) must be in remission from psychogenic polydipsia for at least 24 months and fully understand the nature of his or her co-occurent problems (psychiatric and polydipsia). The client must be willing to engage in outpatient group counseling regarding the ongoing problems that arise in daily living and understand the cyclic nature of addictive behavior.

A candidate ready for discharge to a SIL unit will have a predischarge conference with the aforementioned personnel in attendance (see Admission Criteria) providing feedback regarding the individual's strengths and needs. Quantitative and qualitative data will be reviewed in the psychiatric and functional domains to provide support for the potential discharge. If the committee members are in agreement, a preadmission six-week trial will be arranged with the receiving agency representatives present. The rationale for the eight-week duration is because of the "honeymoon effect" on the candidate living with greater independence. The extended time period allows any concerns to be addressed that routinely arise under these new living arrangements. It also facilitates quicker intervention by the outreach team if the candidate is deemed "going off the rails," ostensibly relapsing, and requires a quick transfer to the former housing arrangement, or to the crisis respite resources (CRR).

The outreach team should also be apprised and act in a liaison capacity to the new, less structured living accommodation in a setting such as SIL or the more structured group home if the client has relapsed. It is important to be completely transparent regarding the client's particular needs in regard to optimizing a success built around transitioning to a new living environment. As mentioned above, an eight-week trial period should be invoked if the client is being discharged to a reduced level of care such as a SIL unit. In this instance, the client will be living independently with outreach support staff visiting at regular intervals, initially throughout the week, then, with time, on a more irregular basis. Visual inspections of the living environment, assessment of the client's functioning, and a debriefing with the SIL manager will be made regularly to minimize any failure.

The outreach team will be the client's conduit to the group home continuum while living in a SIL environment. Weekly meetings, then more protracted debriefing with the SIL manager, will include recommendations regarding any changes in the client's therapeutic care. If the client fails to complete the eight-week trial period at the SIL location, the client will be returned immediately to the RTH group home from whence they came and reenter the original treatment program, and the process for eventual discharge is repeated.

4. Supported Independent Living Accommodation (SIL)

Facility

The supported independent living accommodation (SIL) is the final link in the group home continuum. This facility is a two-bedroom apartment or semi-detached accommodation in which the client lives and participates in daily outpatient activities. The ideal candidate for this living environment is a higher functioning individual diagnosed with schizophrenia, schizoaffective disorder, or one of the AXIS II diagnoses, stabilized and compliant with following a medication protocol. The client has a conceptual understanding of psychogenic polydipsia and has increased control over seeking out and overdrinking any/all fluids. Where can such an ideal candidate be found among the many available clients housed in the other residential resources? A good question with hopefully a cogent response.

Admission Criteria

The selection of a candidate to live in a supported independent accommodation is a steady, methodical, and meticulous process usually hampered by politics, pressure groups, and the candidate's own inclinations to "get out on my own." Without reiterating the previous group home's admission criteria, it must be emphatically stated that this particular treatment facility is the most prone to resident relapse and requires close perusal, albeit from a distance, if that contradiction can be understood.

The client's first six weeks settling in without in-house staff are the most precarious and precipitate the highest frequency of relapse. More specifically, the responsibility of overseeing the client's care falls on the SIL manager and outreach team, who work in tandem. The SIL manager pops in during the first six weeks, on a daily or twice daily basis, to interact with the client and meet the client's numerous, instrumental requests (e.g., fixing appliances, television, computer, windows, toilet, drapes, household chores, etc.,).

The outreach team, in regular contact with the SIL manager (e.g., daily) meets face to face with the client in the facility a minimum of semiweekly (i.e., 12 times in six weeks), to evaluate the client's status with outpatient structured activities, household chores and medication compliance.

 If the client fulfills the six-week trial period, a decision will be made by the outreach team and SIL manager, in consultation with the director of residential services, about the gradual titration of service provision by the outreach team, for the client.

A client who begins to falter and is showing signs of being unable to cope in a semi-independent living environment (regardless of the period in the SIL environment), is relocated to the most available bed in the RTH group home or the crisis respite resources (CRR). This point cannot be overemphasized!

Staffing Model

The staffing model consists of the outreach team, the SIL manager and other disciplines brought in to facilitate problem resolution. Initially, there is a lot of communication with the director of residential services, which over time is reduced in frequency, to coincide with the client's improvement in living skills and adapting to more freedom of movement (e.g., no curfews).

Outreach Team

As mentioned earlier in the chapter, one of the functions of the outreach team is to increase client comfort when transitioning from one facility to another throughout the treatment continuum. It is an especially important role for this particular living accommodation, being the final leg in the client's journey toward responsible drinking behavior and successfully coping with emotional problems.

Unfortunately, because psychogenic polydipsia is a co-occurent disorder, usually combined with schizophrenia, and also a traded addiction (e.g., alcohol), the road to treatment success is often wrought with day-to-day coping problems. If these problems are not addressed quickly, they can lead to relapse and the demise of the placement. In these circumstances the client can be in denial and rationalize with the outreach team that the lapse in judgement was a "one-off" and will not happen again— "please give me another chance"—and the cycle begins again.

Pride aside, the outreach team should carefully assess the situation and discuss the treatment status and client disposition with the director of residential services face to face if possible.

The majority of the time, precursor stressors that have been unresolved by the client are the culprit, thus causing the relapse, and should be identified by the outreach team. Attempts to rectify them should be made quickly and effectively. In the meantime, the director of residential services should be kept in the loop and alternative living options (e.g., crisis respite resources) made available.

SIL Manager

The supported independent living accommodation manager should, with the support of the outreach team, become an important conduit in the treatment success of the client. More specifically, regular, routine household checks (e.g., daily to twice weekly) will identify any instrumental problems presented by the client. For example, a pattern of poor cleaning and dishwashing, personal care problems, incomplete laundry, furniture breakage, inappropriate foodstuffs, and delinquent friends (and the list goes on) will provide and substantiate the more intimate, underlying emotional problems that are occurring with the client. It is recommended that the SIL manager have an in-depth understanding of the nature of this clinical population and be able to communicate in such a way as to minimize a threat being implied by the manager's presence with the client.

This is not as easy as it sounds, as clients diagnosed with psychogenic polydipsia are most often schizophrenic, which, by the very nature of its presenting features, challenges interpersonal relationships from being formed easily. It takes a long time for a feeling of comfort and trust to be formed into a perceived caring alliance with the SIL manager, if it comes at all. The following steps will help reduce communication problems.

At the outset of the placement, the outreach team, the client, and the SIL manager should discuss the nature of the manager's role to reduce any misunderstandings about the manager's comings and goings at the client's living accommodation. The client is given a written handout of all of the tasks germane to the manager's job of overseeing the living accommodation on a day-to-day basis. The client is also informed in writing that any problems in the facility are expected to result in immediate contact with the SIL manager, and failure to do so could have serious consequences regarding the client's tenancy. The client is also informed that the outreach team is as close as the telephone or email if any communication problems occur with the SIL manager, and that contact is expected to be initiated by the client. Over a period of time (i.e., several months) a workable and less stressful relationship should develop between the SIL manager and the client.

Treatment Program

The client will continue with the outpatient programs developed in the RTH group home. The Outreach Team will monitor the client's continued involvement in these programs and liaise with the respective program personnel as required. As time progresses and successes are achieved, the client's outpatient program will be adjusted with new programs to replace those programs that are completed, increasing the client's repertoire of life skills.

The outreach team and the client can review the outpatient treatment plan at any time to assess the level of success (i.e., learning curve) and make adjustments as required, to maximize growth of knowledge. Once again, input from any resources in the group home continuum and outpatient programs may be brought in and pooled to facilitate treatment progress.

A frequent question asked is, "When if ever will the client be able to live on his/her own?" From the writer's experience with this clinical population, the chances of living alone successfully without professional support is a metaphoric loaded gun to the head.

The research articles detailed earlier in Chapter Two do mention success stories over a limited period of time (e.g., 12 months), but seldom, if ever, is there a cure or at least a marked reduction in level of fluid consumption so as to forgo professional support over an extended period of time. The interaction between schizophrenic symptoms—the reduced level of self-awareness due to frontal lobe impairment and the relapsing-remitting course of psychogenic polydipsia—is a perplexing, unrelenting problem to treat.

However, optimism is an important ingredient for any treatment success and with time new treatment approaches may find a way to better effect change with clients diagnosed with this co-occurring disorder.

5. Crisis Respite Resources (CRR)

Facility and Staffing

The crisis respite resources unit (CRR) is located within one of the group homes of the continuum and is specifically developed to be utilized in times of emergency. One to three beds will be sequestered and made available during crisis periods, which usually last less than two weeks (e.g., discharge from SIL). This unit is comprised of members from the outreach team, who rotate their role as external liaison workers to that of inpatient crisis workers on a shift basis, as scheduled. It is important to note that this emergency service is a unit located within a group home of the continuum (e.g., PAIT; SRTGH; RTH), but is not to be compromised—that is, borrowing its staff or resources for other treatment purposes!

The treatment course of psychogenic polydipsia is a long and arduous one, fraught with client problems and staffing difficulties in managing this clinical population. If the group home continuum has approximately 25 clients at any time, it is imperative a crisis service be attached to the treatment program. It will be utilized!

Admission Criteria
A decision is made by the group home staff and/or the outreach team, in consultation with the director of residential services, that the bed is to be utilized until the crisis is resolved. If there is more than one crisis occurring, requiring more than one bed during the interim, upon the discretion of the director of residential services, another open bed may be sequestered from another group home in the continuum. It is therefore important, if possible, to have up to three beds made available as emergent beds located on the same unit. Emergency services designated to one group home in the continuum reduces confusion and increases the legitimacy of this much needed resource.

Discharge Criteria
When the crisis is deemed resolved by the director of residential services, the client is returned to his or her original living accommodation. The crisis bed(s) are for short term only and should only be used for this purpose.

Treatment Program
The outreach team members will oversee the client's recovery by identifying the precipitating events that influenced the crisis. Most common are the client's noncompliance with medication and relapsing to overdrinking any/all fluids. Other influencing stressors might be: adjustment problems emanating from the environment, outpatient programs, and the client's living accommodation (e.g., household chores neglected); family problems that impinge on the client's emotional ambiance (e.g., rumination about the problem); ambivalence about self-worth and a tendency to self-medicate to reduce stress; social isolation, resulting in a lack of social support and reassurance that could ease the anxiety felt by the client; and fear of the future—the greater the extent to which things are unknown, the greater facility there is for speculation of a fearful kind.

Generally, effective management of anxiety facilitates a client's physical recoveries, enabling coping strategies to be learned, which include cognitive behavioral therapy (e.g., challenging automatic thoughts), progressive deep muscle relaxation, thought stopping, counting while visualizing numbers to interfere with emotional arousal, and diaphragmatic breathing. Effective management of anxiety also increases the client's capacity to attend, concentrate, memory retrieve, and problem solve. The client with a co-occurrent disorder tends to view physicians, therapists, and nurses as powerful authorities who are in control. The client in crisis often verbalizes a "one-down" position from the authority figures.

Unfortunately, in the context of having a serious combined problem, the crisis reinforces and exacerbates a lack of self-assertion and problem-solving ability. In conjunction, a previous history of challenging authority figures who "chastised" the client for overdrinking any/all fluids may lead the individual to feel particularly vulnerable to rejection or abuse by those with power. What fuels the crisis in these situations is a typical reaction of reticence or failure to seek help, disagreeing with suggestions, or seeking alternate resources to resolve the problem for fear of "bothering" the caseworker and risking retaliation or criticism. This weighs heavily with a client diagnosed with schizophrenia whose stress threshold is at a vulnerable level.

Therapeutic Strategies for Crisis Intervention

Once outreach team members are involved, they must listen to the client. Listening communicates caring and interest by the crisis worker. Secondly, it allows the client to unburden by verbalizing the stressor, which, when spoken aloud, heard, and reevaluated by the outreach worker, offers a more realistic interpretation of the event. An anxious client benefits from the repeated reassurance and evidence that the crisis team is concerned and caring and will not abandon or deceive the client. Such support should be expressed both directly, in a warm and accepting manner, and indirectly, by attention and responsiveness to the client's needs.

Complicated information, or information that might be perceived as psychologically threatening, should not be given just once but explained on several occasions and, if required, in several different ways. Clients should then be asked to "replay" the information and to question anything with which they disagree or about which they are suspicious. This method of intervention helps to assure that the clients hear what is being said and question any areas of confusion. Clients in crisis have reduced concentration, listening skills, and adequate recall of information and are thus likely to distort facts in accord with their concerns and fears.

During the crisis episode and subsequently, the client should be praised and reinforced for confronting aspects of the stressor(s) without excessive fear and for showing increased emotional control and calm. Such praise will increase the likelihood of desirable behaviors recurring and contribute to the client's self-esteem. More specifically, thinking of oneself positively as being increasingly relaxed helps to build self-confidence and contributes to further calm and the reduction in anxiety-related behaviors. This is an important factor, as a client diagnosed with psychogenic polydipsia tends to seek out and overdrink any/all fluids when stressed. As a result and stated earlier in this section, time should be set aside for the client to learn and practice successful coping strategies, such as diaphragmatic breathing and progressive deep muscle relaxation techniques which relax specific muscle groups. These exercises can help reduce body tension and associated feelings of anxiety, as well as help stabilize mood.

Lastly, it is important to set small but attainable goals. This stepwise, shaping approach stimulates optimal motivation for both the client and the crisis team because it allows frequent, fairly immediate successes while avoiding the frustration and demoralization of failure or of excessively delayed success. With the abatement of the crisis, the client is capable of returning to the previous living accommodation and lifestyle. The goal of the coping strategies is not to make the client totally free of stress—characteristically, that rarely happens with this clinical population—but rather to moderate stress and provide the client with an increased armamentarium to reduce needless relapses in the future.

REFERENCES

Ashby, Y. (1987). Planned change: The development of a program for the management of self induced water intoxication. *Canadian Journal of Psychiatric Nursing*, 28(1), 12-14.Bachrach, L. (1992). Psychosocial rehabilitation and psychiatry in the care of long-term patients. *American Journal of Psychiatry*, 149, 1455-63.

Baier, M., & Gaertner, J. (1991). Target weight procedure: Preventing water intoxication. *Journal of Psychosocial Nursing Mental Health Services,* 29(11), 5-9.

Barahal, H.S. (1938). Water intoxication in a mental case. *Psychiatric Quarterly*, 12, 767-771.

Baumeister, A.A., & Zaharia, E.S. (1987). Withdrawal and commitment of basic care staff in residential programs. In S. Landesman & P. Vietze (Eds.), *Living environments and mental retardation* (pp. 229-267). Washington, DC: American Association on Mental Retardation.

Beasley, J., Krol, J., & Sovner, R. (1992). Community-based crisis mental health services for persons with developmental disabilities: the S.T.A.R.T. model. *The Habilitative Mental Healthcare Newsletter*, 11, 55-58.

Bernstein, G.S., Ziarnik, J.P., Rudrud, E.H & Czajkowski, L.A. (1981). *Behavioral habilitation through proactive programming*. Baltimore, MD: Paul H. Brookes.

Bowen, L., Glynn, S.M., & Marshall, B.D., Kurth, C.L & Hayden, J.L. (1990).Successful behavioral treatment of polydipsia in a schizophrenic patient. *Journal of Behavioral Therapy in Experimental Psychiatry*, 21, 53-61.

Boyd, M.A., Williams, L., Evenson, R., Eckert, Beaman, M., & Carr, T.R. (1992). Target weight procedure for disordered water balance in long-term care facilities. *Journal of Psychosocial Nursing*, Vol. 30, No. 12.

Bremner, A.J., & Regan, A (1991). Intoxicated by water. Polydipsia and water intoxication in a mental handicap hospital. *British Journal of Psychiatry*, 158, 244-250.

Brooker, C., Falloon, I., Goldberg, D., Graham-Hole, V., & Hillier, V. (1994). The outcome of training community psychiatric nurses to deliver psychosocial intervention. *British Journal of Psychiatry*, 165, 199-204.

Cochrane, B.A., Goering, P., Durbin, J. et al. (2000). Tertiary mental health services: 11.Sub-populations and best practices for service delivery. *Canadian Journal of Psychiatry*, Vol. 45(3).

Coleman, J.C & Paul, G.L (2001). Relationship between staffing ratios and effectiveness of inpatient psychiatric units. *Psychiatric Services,* Vol. 52, No. 10, 1374-1379.

Cosgray, M.A., Davidhizar, R., Newman, G., & Kreisl, R (1993). A program for water-intoxicated patients at a state hospital. *Clinical Nurse Specialist*, Vol. 7, No. 2.

Cosgray, R., Hanna, V., Davidhizar, R., & Smith, J. (1990). The water-intoxicated patient. *Archives of Psychiatric Nursing*, 4(5), 308-312.

Costanzo, E.S., Antes, L.M., & Christensen, A.J. (2004). Behavioral and medical treatment of chronic polydipsia in a patient with schizophrenia and diabetes insipidus. *Psychosomatic Medicine*, 66, 283-286.

Cullen, H., Hlagi, J., & Godin, K. paper (August, 2001). Adult Residential Treatment(A.R.T) Quality Improvement Project – H3A Redevelopment Project. *Riverview Psychiatric Hospital*. Coquitlam, BC, Canada.

Davidson, P.W., Cain, N.N., Sloane-Reeves, J.E., et al. (1995). Crisis intervention for community-based individuals with developmental disabilities and behavioral and psychiatric disorders. *Mental Retardation*, 33, 21-30.

Delva, N.J., & Crammer, J.L. (1988). Polydipsia in chronic psychiatric patients: Body weight and plasma sodium. *British journal of Psychiatry*, 152, 242-245.

Dixon, T.P., Goll, s., & Stanton, K.M. (1988). Case management issues and practices in head injury rehabilitation. *Rehabilitation Counseling Bulletin*, 31, 325-343.

Eastern Oregon Human Services Consortium (2010). *Residential Group Homes Continuum*. State-wide Residential Resources in Oregon.

Essocks, S., Hargreaves, W.A., & Dohm, F.A. (1996). Clozapine eligibility among state hospital patients. *Schizophrenia Bulletin* 22, 15-25.

Evans, R.W. & Preston, B.K. (1990). Day rehabilitation programming: A theoreticalmodel. In J. S. Keutzer & P. Wehman, *Communtiy Integration Following Traumatic Brain Injury*. Baltimore: Paul. H. Brookes.

Frank, R.G., & Brookmeyer. R. (1995). Managed mental health care and patterns of inpatient utilization for treatment of affective disorders. *Social Psychiatry Psychiatric Epidemiology*, 30, 220-223.

Gardner, W., & Hunter, R.H. (2003). Psychosocial Diagnosis and Treatment Services inIn-patient Psychiatric Facilities For Persons With Mental Retardation: Practice Guides. *Mental Health Aspects of Developmental Disabilities,*Vol. 6, No. 2.

Gibson, M.C. (2010). Psychogenic polydipsia. WikiDoc Resources.Godleski, L.S., Vieweg, W.V.R., Leadbetter, R.A., Hundley, P.L., Harrington, D.P., & Harrington, D.P. (1989). Day-to-day care of chronic schizophrenic patients subject to water intoxication. *Annals of Clinical Psychiatry*, 1, 179-185.

Goldman, M.B., & Luchins, D. J. (1987). Prevention of episodic water intoxication with target weight procedure. *American Journal of Psychiatry*, 144, 367-366.

Gossett, J., Lewis, J., & Barnhart, D. (1983). *To Find a Way. The Outcome of Hospital Treatment of Disturbed Adolescents*. New York: Brunner/Mazel.

Gurel, L. (1964). *Correlates of psychiatric hospital effectiveness, in symposium: An assessment of psychiatric hospital effectiveness*. Proceedings of the American Psychological Association convention, Los Angeles, Washington, DC

H3A Treatment Team – Research Study (June, 2001). Research Study Summary: Self Induced Water Intoxication (SIWI) Ward – Adult Residential Transfer Program Redevelopment Project. *Riverview Psychiatric Hospital*. Coquitlam, BC, Canada.

Harisprasad, M,K., Eisinger, R.P., & Nadler, R.M et al. (1988). Hyponatremia in psychogenic polydipsia. *Archives of Internal Medicine*, 140, 1639-1642.

Hastings, M. Correspondence (October 4, 2001). Alberta Hospital Treatment Program, Ponoka, *Alberta, Canada. Alberta Mental Health Board – Alberta Hospital Ponoka Site*.

Held, T. (1995). *Schizophreniebehandlung in der Familie. Eine Kontrollierte Studie zur Wirsamkeit familiarer Verhaltenstherapie bei der Ruckfallprophylaxe schizophrenerErkrankungen*. Frankfurt am Main: Perter Lang.

Hembree, W.E. (1985, July/August). Getting involved: Employees as case managers. *Business and Health Week*, pp. 11-14.

Hershen, M., & Barlow, D.H. (1976). *Single case experimental designs: Strategies for studying behavior change*. New York: Pergamon Press.

Homme, L., Csanyi, A.P.K., Gonzales, M.A., & Rechs, J.R. (1969). *How to use contingency contracting in the classroom*. Champaign, IL: Research Press.

Hoskins, R.G. (1933). Schizophrenia from the physiologicasl point of view. *Annalsof Internal Medicine*, 7, 445-456.

Hutcheon, D. (2003). East Lawn Building – Psychogenic Polydipsia "Water Ward"(2002 – 2003) Annual Report. *Riverview Psychiatric Hospital*, Coquitlam, BC, Canada.

Huxley, N.A., Rendall, M., & Sederer, L. (2000). Psychosocial treatments in schizophrenia: a review of the past 20 years. *Journal of Nervous and Mental Disease* 2000, 188, 187-201.

Jose, C., & Perez-Cruet, J. (1979). Incidence and morbidity of self-induced waterintoxication in state hospital patients. *American Journal of Psychiatry*. 136(2), 221-222.

Keller, F.S (1969). *Learning: Reinforcement theory*. (2nd ed.). New York: Random House.

Kenyon, D.A. (May, 1997). *Strategic Planning With The Hoshin Process*. Quality Digest U.S.A.

Klonoff, E.A., & Morre, D.J. (1984). Compulsive polydipsia presenting as diabetesinsipidus: A behavioral approach. *Journal of Behavioral Therapeutics and Experimental Psychiatry*, 15, 353-358.

Knight, R.C., Weitzer, W.H., & Zimring, C.M. (Eds.). (1978). *Opportunity for control and the built environment: the ELEMR Project*. Amherst, MA: The Environmental Institute, University of Massachusetts.

Koczapski, A.B., & Millson, R.C. (1989). Individual differences in the serum sodium levels in schizophrenic men with self-induced water intoxication. *American Journal of Psychiatry*, 146, 1614-1615.

Koczapski, A.B. Ibraheem, S., Ashby Y.T, et al. (1987). Early diagnosis of water Intoxication by monitoring diurnal variations in body weight (letter). *American Journal of Psychiatry*, 44, 1626.

Koczapski, A, Ibraheem, S, & Paredes, J, et al. (1985) Diurnal variations in hyponatremia and body weight in chronic schizophrenics with self-induced water intoxication. *American Journal of Psychiatry*, 146, 1614-1615.

Kopleowicz, A., Liberman, R.P., & Zarate, R. (2002). Psychosocial treatments for schizophrenica. In: Nathan PE, Gorman, J.M., Eds. *A guide to treatments that work*, 2nd ed. London: Oxford University Press, 201-228.

Landesman, S. (1988). Preventing "institutionalziation" in the community. In M.P. Landesman-Dwyer (Ed.) (1981). Living in the community. *American Journal of Mental Deficiency*, 86, 223-234.

Landesman-Dwyer, S. (1984). Friendships and social behavior. In J. Wortis (Ed.). *Mental retardation and developmental disabilities: An annual review* (Vol. 13, pp. 129-154). New York: Plenum Press.

Landesman-Dwyer, S. (1984b). Residential environments and the social behavior of handicapped individuals. In M. Lewis (Ed.). *Beyond the dyad* (pp. 299-322). New York: Plenum Press.

Landesman-Dwyer., S., & Berkson, G. (1984). Friendships and social behavior. In J. Wortis (Ed.), *Mental retardation and developmental disabilities: An annual review.* (Vol. 13, pp. 129-154). New York: Plenum Press. Lapierre, E., Berthot, B., Gurvitch, M., Rees, I., & Kirch, D. (1990). Polydipsia andhyponatremia in psychiatric patients: Challenge to creative nursing care. *Archives of Psychiatric Nursing.* 4(2), 87-92.

Lasky, D.I, & Dowling, M. (1971). The release rates of state mental hospitals as related to maintenance costs and patient-staff ratio. *Journal of Clinical Psychology,* 27, 272-277.

Leadbetter, R., & Shutty, M., Higgins, P.B., & Pavalonis, D. (1994). Multidisciplinary approach to psychosis, intermittent hyponatremia, and polydipsia. *Schizophrenia Bulletin.* Vol. 20, No. 2.

Ledochowski. M., Kahler, M., Diensil, F.F., Hacker, W., & Barnes, C. (1988). Waterintoxication, the course of an acute schizophrenic experience. *Intensive Care Medicine* 12(1), 47-55.

Leiberman, R.P, & Phipps, C.C. (1987). Innovative treatment and rehabilitation techniques. In W.W Menninger & G. Hannah (Eds). *The chronic mental patient* 11. Washington, DC: American Psychiatric Press: 121-134.

Liberman, R., & Marshall. B. (1993). Polydipsia and hyponatremia. *Hospital and Community Psychiatry,* 44, 184.

Links, S.P., Kirkpatrick, H, & Whelton, C. (1994). Psychosocial rehabilitation and the role of the psychiatrist. *Psychosocial Rehabilitation Journal* 18, 121-129.

Linn, L.S. (1970). State hospital environment and rates of patient discharge. *Archives of General Psychology,* 23, 346-351. Linn, L.S. (1970b). Measuring the effectiveness of mental hospitals. *Hospital and Community Psychiatry* 21, 381-386.

Lundin, R.W. (1974). *Personality: A behavioral analysis.* (2nd ed.). New York: Macmillan.

Lyons, J.S., O'Mahoney, M.T., Miller, S.I., Neme, J., Kabat, J., & Miller, F. (1997). Predicting readmission to the psychiatric hospital in a managed care environment; Implications for quality indicators. *American Journal of Psychiatry,* 154, 337-340.

Mapes, R.E.A & Clarke, M.J. (1975). A path analytic model of psychiatric hospital performance. *Social Science and Medicine* 9, 257-262.

McGorry, P.(2005). Royal Australian and New Zealand College of Psychiatrists clinical practice guidelines for the treatment of schizophrenia and related disorders. *Australianand New Zealand Journal of Psychiatry,* 39, 1-30.

McNally, R., Calamari, J., Hansen, P., et al: (1988). Behavioral treatment of psychogenicPolydipsia. *Journal of Behavioral Experimental Psychiatry*, 19, 57-61.

Menditto, A.A. (2002). A social-learning approach to the rehabilitation of individuals with severe mental disorders who reside in forensic facilities. *Psychiatric Rehabilitation.*Vol. 6, No. 1, 73-93.

Miller, W.R. (1936) Psychogenic factors in the polyuria of schizophrenia. *Journal of Nervous and Mental Disease,* 84, 418.

Moores, B., & Grant, G.W.B. (1977). The "avoidance" syndrome in hospitals for the mentally handicapped. *International Journal of Nursing Studies*, 134, 91-95.

Nadler, D.A. & Tushman, M.L (1988). *Strategic Organization Design: Concepts, Tools, and Processes.* United States of America: Harper Collins Publishers.

Pavalonis, D., Shutty, M., Hundley, P, Leadbetter, R., Vieweg, W., & Downs, M. (1992). Behavioral intervention to reduce water intake in the syndrome of psychosis, intermittent hyponatremia, and polydipsia. *Journal of Behavior Therapeutic Experimental Psychiatry*, 23, 51-57.

Paul, G.L., (2000). Evidence-based practices in inpatient and residential facilities. *Clinical Psychologist* 53(3), 3-11.

Paul, G.L (1986). Net relative cost of the maximum potential utility paradigm. In G.L.Paul (Ed.). *Principles and methods to support cost-effective quality operations: Assessment in Residential Treatment Settings: Part 1.* Champaign, IL, Research Press.

Paul G.L., & Lentz, R.J (1977). *Psychosocial treatment of chronic mental patients.* Cambridge, Mass. Harvard University Press.

Pazaratz, D., Randall, D., Spekkens, J.F., Lazor, A., & Morton, W.J.l. (2000). The four-phase system: A multi-agency coordinated service for very disturbed adolescents. *Residential Treatment for Children and Youth*, 17, 31- 48.

Pfister, H.O. (1934). Disturbances of the autonomic nervous system in schizophrenia and their relations to the insulin, cardiazol, and sleep treatments. *American Journal of Psychiatry*, 94 (May Suppl.), 109-118.

Psychosocial Rehabilitation (PSR) (2010). *Principles of Psychosocial Rehabilitation* (PSR). *Canadian Code of Ethics.* PSR Canada

Raskind, Z.M. (1974). Psychosis, polydipsia and water intoxication. Report of a fatalCase. *Archives of General Psychiatry* 30, 112-114.

Reece, E.P. (1966). *The analysis of human operant behavior*. Dubuque, IA: W.M.C. Brown.

Rilling, S., Bebbington, P., & Kuipers, E et al. (2002). Psychological treatments in schizophrenia. I. Meta-analysis of family intervention and cognitive behaviour therapy. *Psychological Medicine*, 32, 763-782.

Rinard, G.(1989). Water intoxication. *American Journal of Nursing*. Dec, 1635-1638.

Rowntree, L.G. (1923). Water intoxication. *Archives of Internal Medicine*. 32, 157-174.Shesser, R., & Smith, M. (1985). Seizures in psychiatric patients. *American Journal ofEmergency Medicine,* 3, 451-458.

Shostack, A.L. (1987). *Group Homes For Teenagers: A Practical Guide*. New York: Human Sciences Press, Inc.

Siegler, E.L., Tamres, D., Berlin, J.A., Allen-Taylor, L., & Strom, B.L. (1995). Risk factors for the development of hyponatremia in psychiatric inpatients. *Archives of Internal Medicine,* 155, 953-957.

Silverstein, S.M., Hitzel, H., & Schenkel, L. (1998). Identifying and addressing cognitive barriers to rehabilitation readiness. *Psychiatric Services* 49, 34-36.

Skinner, B.F. (1953). *Science and Human Behavior*. New York: Macmillan.

Sleeper, F.H., & Jellinek, E.M. (1936). A comparative physiologic, psychologic and psychiatric study of polyuric and nonpolyuric sxhizophrenic patients. *Journal of Nervous and Mental Disease*, 83, 557-563.

Spradlin, W.W. (1985). Psychogenic polydipsia and water intoxication: Concepts that have failed. *Biological Psychiatry*, 20, 1308-1320.

Snider, K., & Boyd, M. (1991). When they drink too much: Nursing interventions for patients with disordered water balance. *Journal of Psychosocial Nursing*. 29(7), 10-16.

Thomas, J.L., Howe, J., Gaudet, A., & Brantley, P.J. (2001). Behavioral treatment of chronic psychogenic polydipsia with hyponatremia: a unique case of polydipsia in a primary care patient with intractable hiccups. *Journal of Behavior Therapy and Experimental Psychiatry*, 32, 241-250.

Travers, R.W.M. (1977). *Essentials of Learning*. New York: Macmillan.

Ullman, L.P. (1967). *Institution and outcome: A comparative study of psychiatric hospitals.* New York, Pergamon.

Verghese, C., De Leon, J., & Josiassen, R. (1996). Problems and progress in the diagnosis and treatment of polydipsia and hyponatremia. *Schizophrenia bulletin*, 22(3), 455-464.

Verghese, C., de Leon, J., & Simpson, G. (1993). Neuroendocrine factors influencing polydipsia in psychiatric patients: an hypothesis. *Neuropsychopharmacology*, 9, 157- 166.

Vieweg, W.V. R. (1996). In D.B. Schnure, & D. G. Kirch (Eds.). Overview of water balance in schizophrenia (pp. 1-42). Washington, DC. *American Psychiatric Press*.

Vieweg, W.V.R., David, J.J., Rowe, W.T., Peach, M.J., Veldhuis, J.D., Kaiser, D.L., Vieweg, W., & Leadbetter, R. (1990). Water intoxication treatment (letter). *Biological Psychiatry*, 28, 829.

Vieweg, W.V.R., David, J.J., Rowe, W.T., Wampler, G.J., Burns, W.J., & Spradlin, W.W. (1985). Death from self-induced water intoxication among patients with schizophrenic disorders. *Journal of Nervous and Mental disease*, 173, 161-165.

Visalli, H.(1997). Developing a best practice model for care of patients with polydipsia. *Journal of Nursing Care Quality*, 12(1), 53-62.

Wasylenki, D., Goering, P., Cochrane, J., Simon, L.J., & Wirth-Cauchon, J.L. (2000). Tertiary mental health services: I. Key concepts. *Canadian Journal of Psychiatry*, 45, 179-184.

Wolfensberger, W. (1972). *The normaliztion principle in human services*. Toronto: National Institute on Mental Retardation.

Wolins, M. (1974). Group care: Friend or Fow. In M.Wolins (Ed.). *Successful group care. Explorations in the powerful environment*. Chicago: Aldine.

REFERENCES

INDEX

CPSIA information can be obtained
at www.ICGtesting.com
Printed in the USA
LVHW100023281021
701735LV00005B/185